Topics in Primary Care Medicine

Edited by Thomas F. Heston

Published in London, United Kingdom

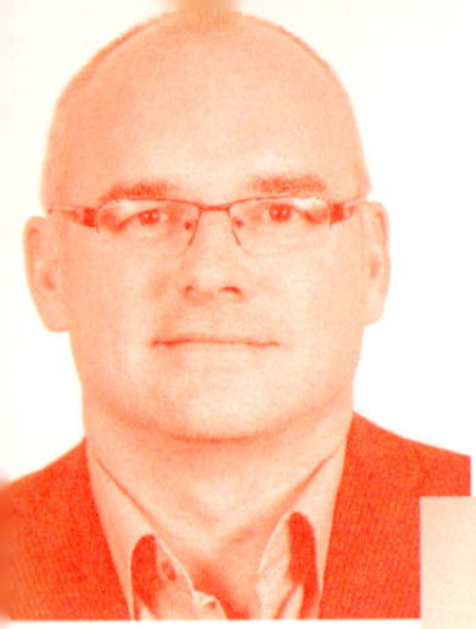
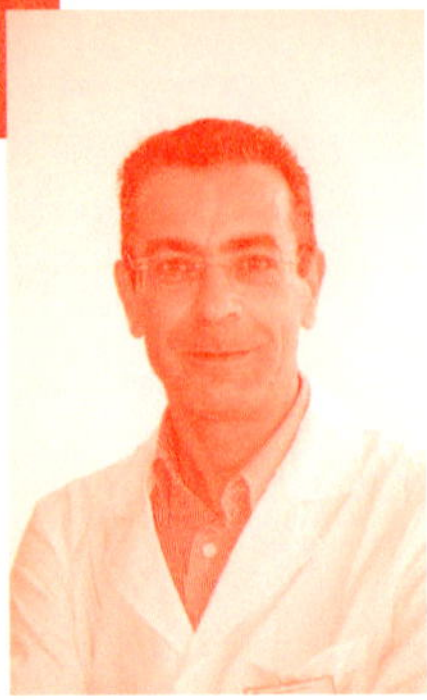
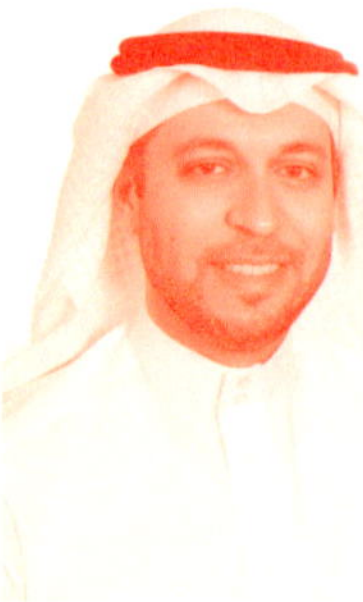
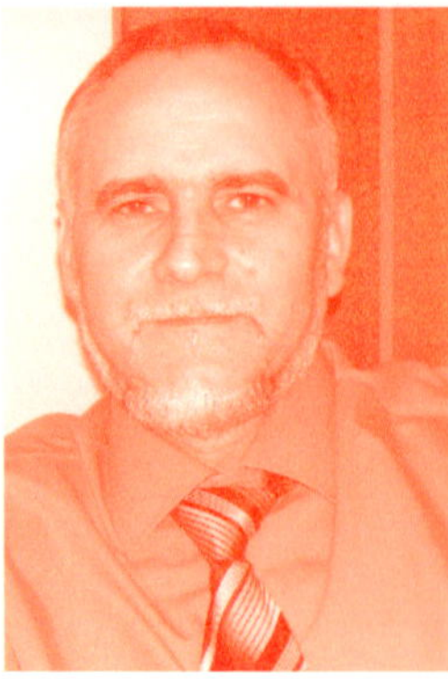
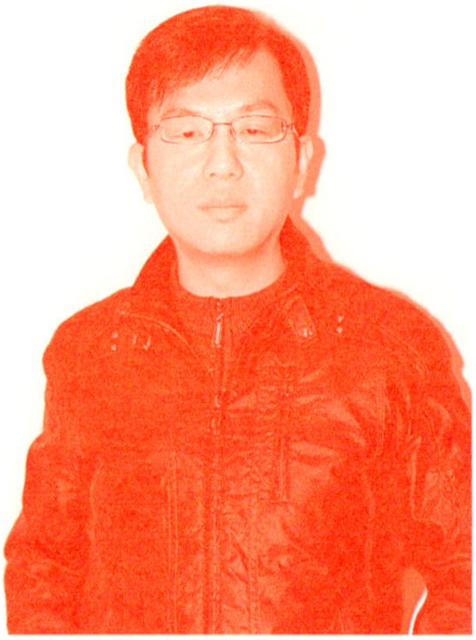
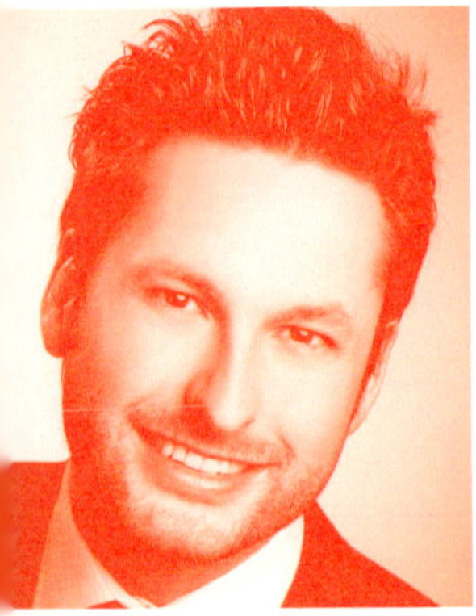
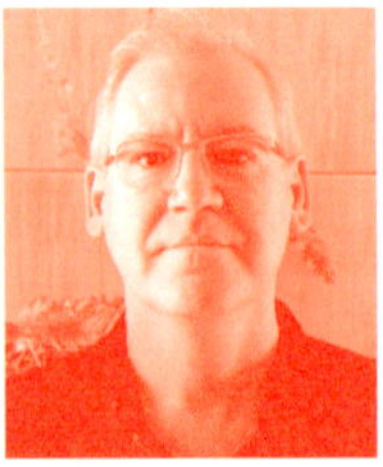

IntechOpen

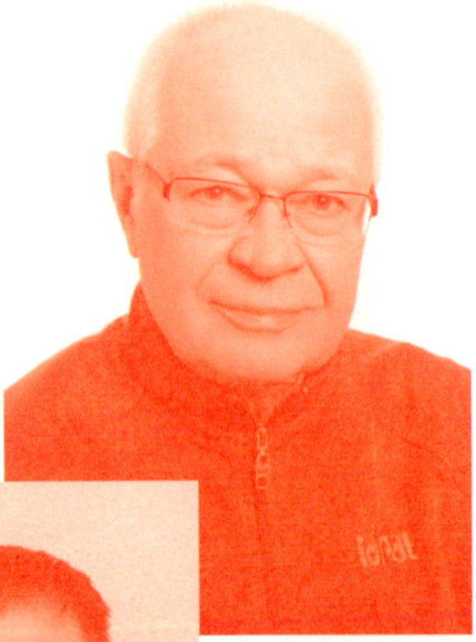
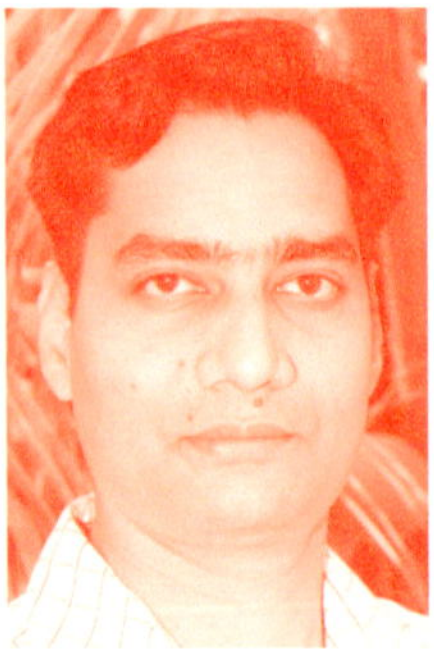
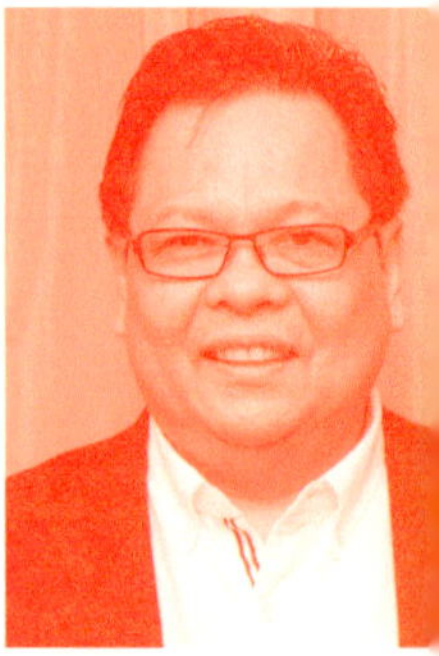
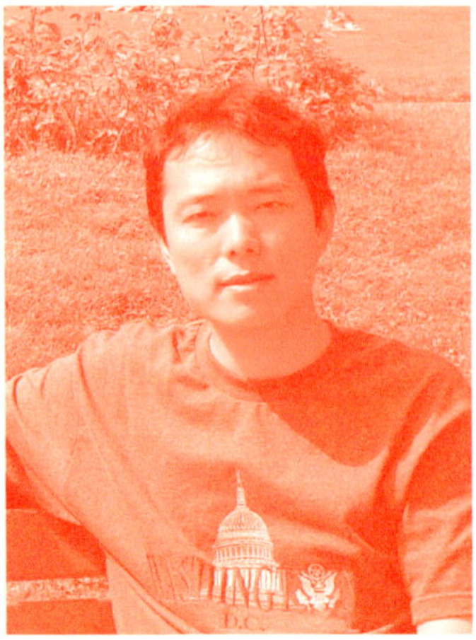
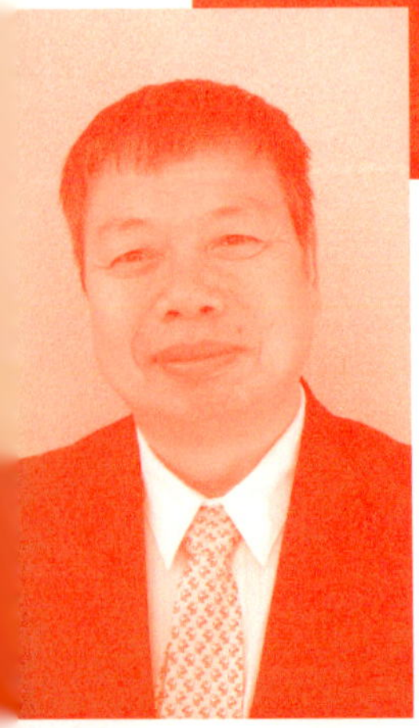
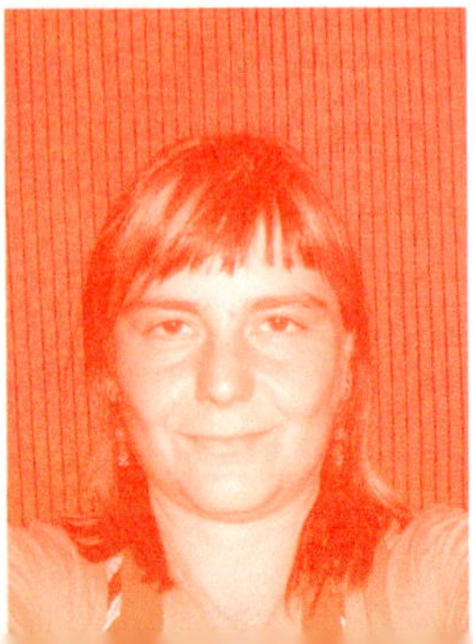

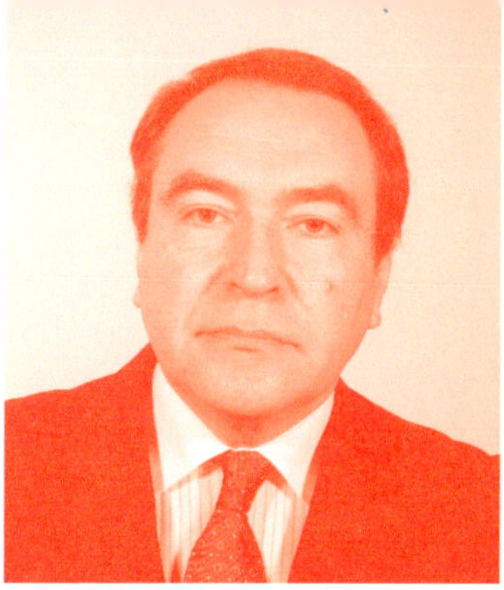

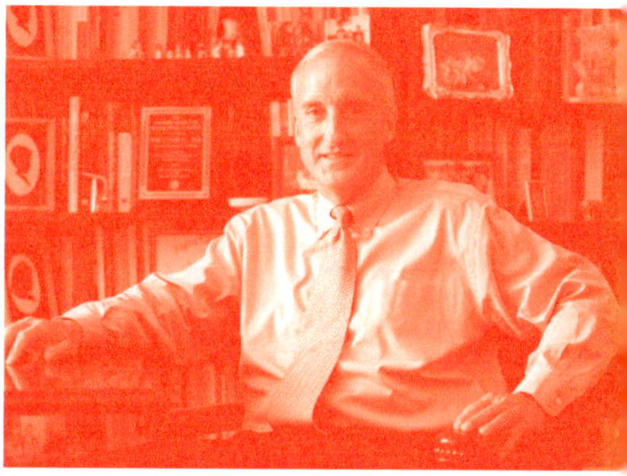

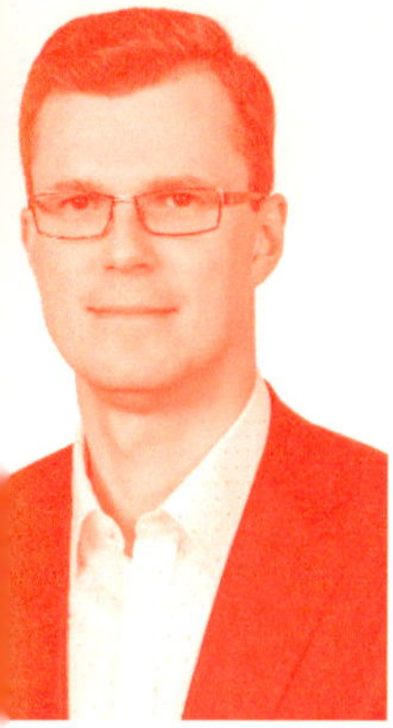

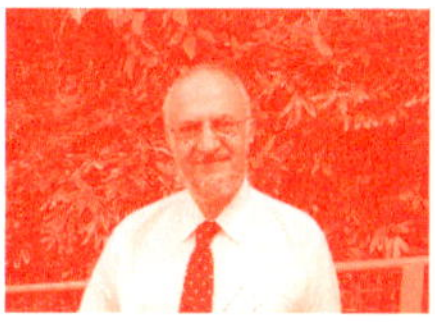

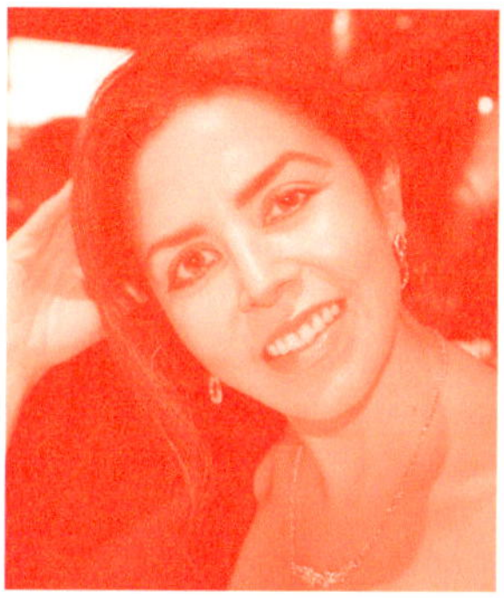

Supporting open minds since 2005

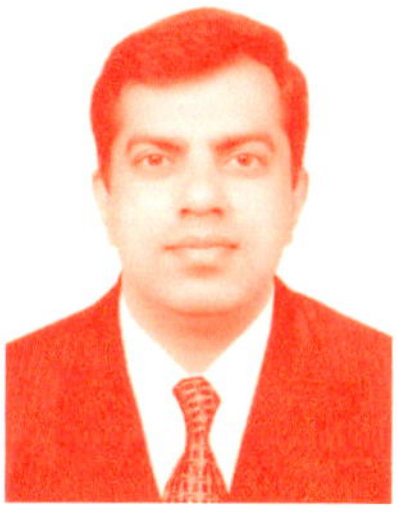

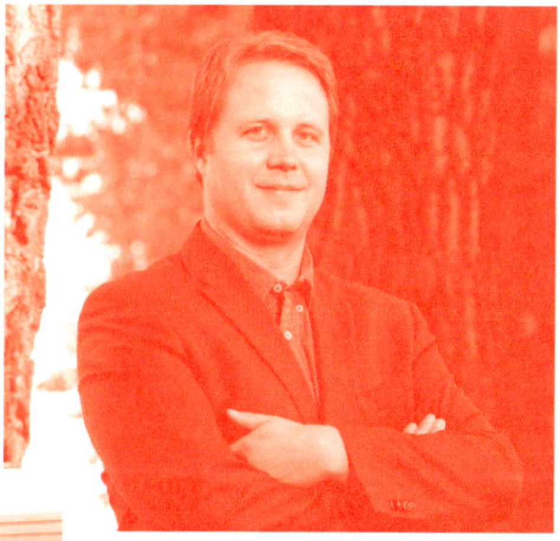

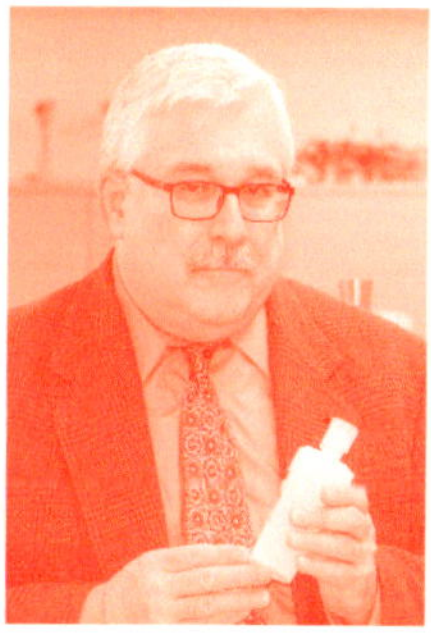

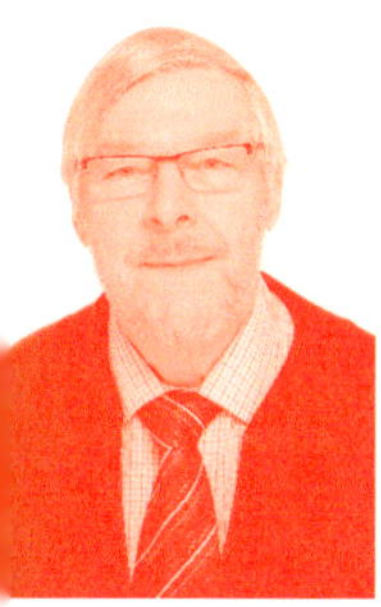

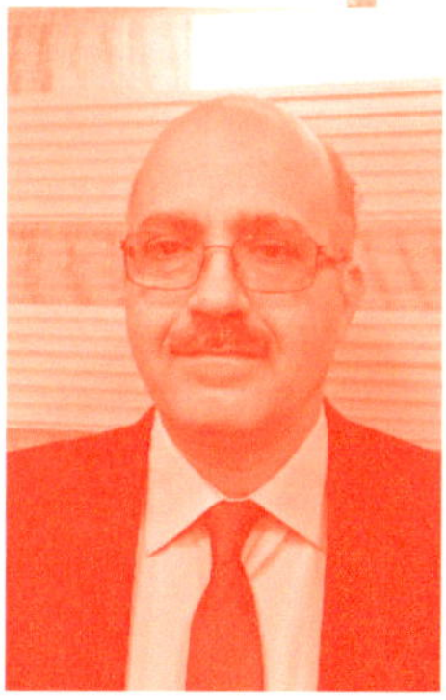

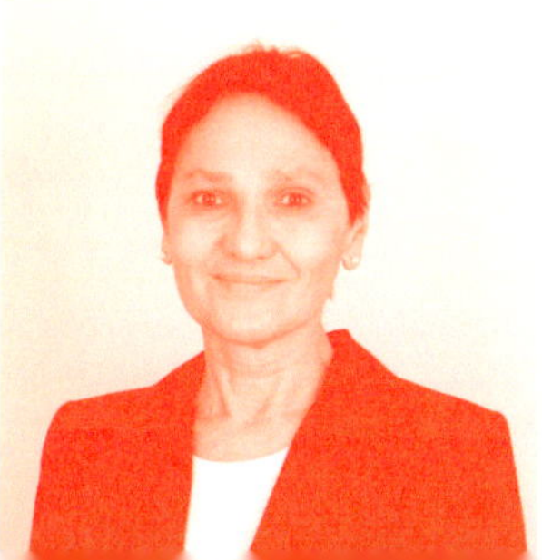

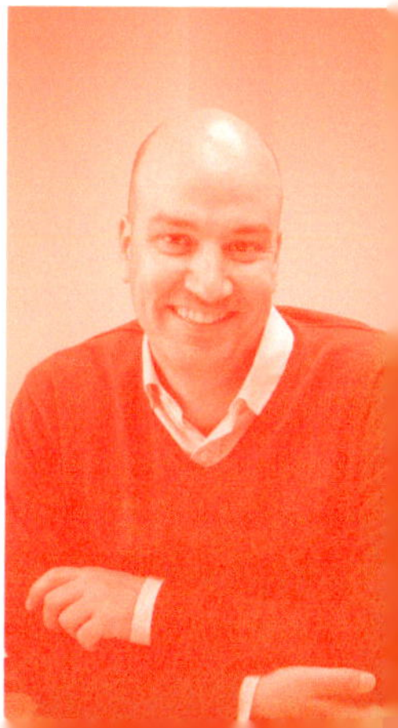

Topics in Primary Care Medicine
http://dx.doi.org/10.5772/intechopen.83135
Edited by Thomas F. Heston

Contributors
Javier Eduardo Escober Torres, Mercedes Libeth Ramos Amador, Jose María Arribas Blanco, Wafa Elgeadi, Belen Chavero, María Alvargonzález Arrancudiaga, Luis Geniz Rubio, Jose Angel Lopez, Sara Alcantara, Macarena Ávila Pérez, Rudika Gmajnic, Stjepan Rudan, Sanda Pribić, Jonathan Comyn Comyn De Rothewelle, Aina Olufemi Odusola, Ayoade Adedokun, Katherine Rowe, Amanda Apple, Fiona McDonald, Abdulnasir Al-Jazairi

First published in London, United Kingdom, 2021 by IntechOpen
IntechOpen is the global imprint of INTECHOPEN LIMITED, registered in England and Wales, registration number: 11086078, 5 Princes Gate Court, London, SW7 2QJ, United Kingdom
Printed in Croatia

British Library Cataloguing-in-Publication Data
A catalogue record for this book is available from the British Library

Additional hard and PDF copies can be obtained from orders@intechopen.com

Topics in Primary Care Medicine
Edited by Thomas F. Heston
p. cm.
Print ISBN 978-1-78985-917-1
Online ISBN 978-1-78985-918-8
eBook (PDF) ISBN 978-1-83880-276-9

For EU product safety concerns:
IN TECH d.o.o., Prolaz Marije Krucifikse Kozulić 3, 51000 Rijeka, Croatia, info@intechopen.com or visit our website at intechopen.com.

Meet the editor

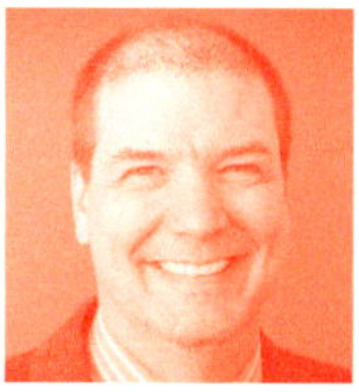

Dr. Thomas F. Heston is a practicing primary care physician and Clinical Associate Professor at the Elson S. Floyd College of Medicine at Washington State University, Spokane, Washington. After graduating from St. Louis University Medical School, St. Louis, Missouri, Dr. Heston went on to do his internship at Duke University, Durham, North Carolina and a residency in Family Medicine at the University of Washington, Seattle, Washington. He has practiced rural family medicine in an underserved region of Idaho and subsequently as a hospitalist physician. He is a fellow of the American Academy of Family Physicians. He has practiced primary care medicine for more than 25 years. His primary research focus is the integration of technology into frontline medicine.

Contents

Preface

Topics in Primary Care Medicine provides readers with an overview of several topics in the broad field of frontline medical care ranging from the treatment of chronic diseases, to the role of surgery in primary care, to a look at patients and physicians in graphical art. The challenges facing primary care clinicians are highly varied, as clinicians in this specialty are responsible for a wide range of knowledge on the fundamental health needs of individuals, families, communities, and the global population. Primary care is rightly called "primary" because it addresses the most basic and fundamental medical needs facing individuals. While no single textbook can address all of these challenges, this book offers an in-depth review of several important topics to enrich readers with a greater understanding of the broad topic of human health and well-being.

Thomas F. Heston, MD, MSc, FAAFP, FASNC, FACNM
Clinical Associate Professor,
Elson S. Floyd College of Medicine,
Washington State University,
Spokane, Washington, USA

Section 1

Primary Care

Chapter 1

Self-Management of Chronic Fatigue Syndrome in Adolescents

Katherine Rowe, Amanda Apple and Fiona McDonald

Abstract

Chronic fatigue syndrome (CFS) or myalgic encephalomyelitis/chronic fatigue syndrome (ME/CFS) is a condition of unknown aetiology that commonly follows an infection. There are no known predictors for recovery or established treatments. At the Royal Children's Hospital (RCH) in Melbourne, Australia, the majority of young people with CFS are provided with symptom management and lifestyle guidance in an outpatient setting. However, for some, educational or social issues preclude progress and for those who request this assistance, since 2012, the Victorian Paediatric Rehabilitation Service has offered an Intensive Self-Management Program. For this program, participants engage in both group and individual sessions, attending 3 days per week for 4 weeks in small groups of 3–4. Interdisciplinary input is from Occupational Therapy, Physiotherapy, Education and Psychology to assist with goal setting and strategies. Outcome measures are obtained at initial assessment, 6 weeks and 6 months post-program. Support is offered for 12 months post-program. For both the outpatient program and the intensive program the outcomes and feedback from patient and family has influenced the approach and focus. This chapter outlines the current approach and how it has evolved over time.

Keywords: adolescent, chronic fatigue syndrome, management, rehabilitation, outcomes

1. Introduction

Chronic fatigue syndrome is a condition of unknown aetiology that commonly follows an infective process in young people. There is a new onset of fatigue for at least 3–6 months that is not relieved by rest and not explained by other medical conditions. Post-exertional malaise, cognitive difficulties and unrefreshing sleep are present. In addition, a variety of somatic symptoms are commonly present such as headache, abdominal or muscle pain, as well as flu-like symptoms without fever, and symptoms associated with orthostatic intolerance [1–5]. The key features and symptom patterns in young people have remained consistent [6–9]. Anxiety and depression may also be present but when compared with population levels, were only mildly increased in prevalence, and generally did not precede the illness. They were understandably associated with diagnosis delay, not being believed or social isolation [8, 10].

There is currently no defined treatment, as the underlying pathology is not well understood [11]. Similarly, there are no known predictors for recovery [10]. When this illness occurs during childhood and adolescence, it is at a period of significant

 IntechOpen

developmental changes. In those that report recovery, the duration of illness has mean of 5 years and range 1–16 years [10]. With long-term follow-up, there is a significant proportion that does not report recovery [10, 12, 13]. There is disruption to their educational, social and physical activities, which create huge challenges for the young people and their families [14, 15]. It is the commonest cause of reduced time at school [16, 17], and has a significant impact on educational functioning [18]. Hence, in addition to managing symptoms, strategies for coping with this chronic illness and its impact on the young person and the family have been central to its management in this clinic [10]. Although there are other chronic illnesses during childhood and adolescence that have physical, emotional, cognitive or educational impacts [19–23], this illness does affect all these areas. Neglecting these aspects can compound the effect of the illness, and impact on the developmental tasks of adolescence or the transition to or from adolescence. Parents have a role in helping navigate these tasks, as well as trying to manage a child who is unwell [19, 20].

This chapter will outline the management strategies that have been employed in an outpatient setting that have been guided by feedback from young people over a period of more than 25 years; a description of the development since 2012 of an intensive self-management program for those who need additional assistance; and observations about characteristics of participants in the program and their reasons for referral.

2. Outpatient management

2.1 Chronic fatigue syndrome outpatient clinic at the Royal Children's Hospital

The Royal Children's Hospital is a specialised secondary and tertiary referral paediatric and adolescent hospital that services metropolitan Melbourne and all rural areas for the state of Victoria including bordering areas in neighbouring states. Furthest distances require 4–5 h of car travel. Referrals are received from family doctors or from specialist paediatricians. Victoria has a population of 6.3 million and is multicultural. There is a universal health system that ensures citizens can access health care free of charge to the family. There is also a private health system that can provide partially subsidised health and allied health care.

The CFS clinic has been functioning since 1989. In the early years of the clinic the Holmes definition and Fukuda criteria for CFS were available [2, 3, 21]. However, acceptance of the diagnosis in young people was uncommon in the medical fraternity. It was well recognised that Epstein Barr Virus (EBV) infection (or glandular fever) could run a prolonged course during adolescence. Irrespective of whether EBV was confirmed, it was assumed in some cases, that this was the cause of these symptoms. Alternative explanations that were entertained were depression, stress, school refusal or somatisation disorder or the possibility of undisclosed family difficulties. Parents who were anxious due to concern about the unexplained change in the young person were often considered to be contributing to their illness. Hence many who attended the clinic had experienced unsatisfying encounters with the medical profession.

The reported symptoms were very consistent among the young people attending. The presence of post-exertional malaise (PEM), unrefreshing sleep, cognitive difficulties, persistent fatigue and pain (headache, muscle, abdominal) were all almost universally reported. Sore throats and lymph nodes, feeling hot and cold and symptoms later recognised as associated with orthostatic intolerance were very common. These symptoms were consistently reported even though at the time there was no access to this information in the public arena.

Although the intravenous immunoglobulin trial in young people appeared a promising treatment [22], trials in adults were inconclusive [23–25], and approval was not granted for its use. Thus options for treatment reverted to general management strategies for chronic illness. We relied on feedback from young people to inform us regarding what was helpful in their management. The service has since expanded to several paediatricians and access to a 4-week self-management program run by the Victorian Paediatric Rehabilitation Service at the hospital.

2.2 Diagnosis

A diagnosis of CFS is made following an extensive history, to confirm the presence of key symptoms, examination and routine investigations to exclude alternative diagnoses. These symptoms include PEM, unrefreshing sleep and cognitive symptoms as well as additional somatic symptoms [15]. Other conditions including school refusal, somatisation disorder, eating disorders, isolated significant depression or anxiety, connective tissue disorders, coeliac disease or endocrine disorders are specifically checked. An adolescent psychosocial (HEADSS) screen is also conducted where appropriate [26]. Passive standing test was not routinely performed initially. However, upon recognition of the association of orthostatic intolerance with ME/CFS this assessment was included [1].

Routine screening investigations included coeliac screen, thyroid function and antinuclear antibody. Serology for EBV or cytomegalovirus (CMV) is routinely assessed or if there was any likelihood of overseas or tropical infections or if the young person had been in areas where Ross River Virus, Q fever (Coxiella burnetti), Barmah forest virus were endemic, serology for exposure is also checked.

2.3 Management

2.3.1 Initial appointment

Following diagnosis, the young person is asked to: rate the most troublesome symptom/s that he/she would like help with; outline his/her aspirations prior to illness; describe current school attendance, interests, and previous participation in sport, the family situation and supports including parental work schedule, and means of transport to school or activities. The young person is provided with a brief explanation of our current knowledge, a plan for managing the most severe symptoms, and an outline of a management plan that the young person would devise.

2.3.2 Management plan designed by the young person

The rationale for the management plan is to minimise the impact of chronic illness while accommodating the specific issues associated with CFS. As CFS affects the educational, physical, social and emotional aspects of their life, it is considered important to not neglect any of these areas. This should include some proactive social contact, academic input, physical activity and a commitment to attend something enjoyable outside of home on a regular basis. None of these activities is to be neglected but the proportion does not have to be equal. The plan needs to be sustainable for at least a month before it is reviewed. For example, some physical activity is required to prevent becoming so de-conditioned that they are unsure whether they are weak and fatigued because they are unwell or because muscles are not being used. Social contact is important to ensure that the social learning that occurs during adolescence (how to respond in different situations, what behaviour is acceptable and how to interpret different social situations and how to understand one's peers) is not neglected. It can be very daunting later when it is expected that these skills have been acquired. Academic engagement is important so that they feel that their life chances have not been destroyed. The regular enjoyable activity outside of home is something that they have chosen to attend because it is 'worth it' and will not result in a prolonged recovery. It removes any prevarication regarding whether they feel well enough, whether they would cope or whether it would be easier not to go. Only if they are unable to move out of bed do they not attend. This hopefully prevents the reluctance to make decisions, to be adventurous or to be reliable.

In addition, young people generally have not had to learn to prioritise their activities during their teenage years but it is needed as developing adults. It is explained that they need to learn this much earlier than most and it is a very useful skill to acquire. Some activities, for example, attending school for an enjoyable subject could fulfil social, academic and enjoyable activities and also require some physical activity. If their important social network was outside of school then there needed to be an effort to engage with that group for a period of time that was manageable. If some young people felt that 'life was not worth living' if they could not play sport, as this was their main social connection, then adjustments could be made. They could be part of the team by 'coming off the bench' for a few minutes or not being required to actively train. They could be moved to a team position that did not require a lot of stamina. On the other hand, for some, physical activity may be a few activities of daily living spaced over the day, or once they are able to do some activity and have increased their strength, they often chose a variety of activities that they enjoy.

Their aspirations (prior to becoming unwell) play a key role in the decisions regarding their education. Attending school for set hours, rather than for specific subjects is difficult to sustain. Reduction in the school subject load to include subjects and teachers they liked, as well as subjects that are pre-requisites for what they want to do as a career is crucial. Trying to keep up with all subjects when only given minimal information is a source of unnecessary stress, and this rarely succeeds. A planned timetable ensures that the arrangements provide some consistency and predictability for the family (and for the teaching staff) and be manageable for the young person. If the symptoms are severe, the extent of 'academic input' may be reduced to reading about a hobby or reading a story that they are already familiar with.

It is explained to the young person that these consequences of illness can be more damaging than the illness itself and can occur with any chronic illness. Neglecting these areas creates significant hurdles to recovery such as: navigating social anxiety and social learning; entering the workforce without a potentially enjoyable, satisfying or more lucrative, less physically demanding job; needing to increase strength, or not having the confidence or resilience to know how they are able to manage their life. The young person is asked to estimate how they can balance these tasks within the bounds of the amount of energy available over the period of a week. The young people make those decisions over the subsequent few weeks and discuss their plan with their parents.

2.3.3 Symptom management

Only the most severe one or two symptoms are treated initially. Often treating one symptom such as sleep disturbance, and allowing them to take control of their life with the management plan reduces the severity of some of the other troublesome symptoms. Despite the prominent fatigue, malaise and concentration difficulties, the complaints of headache and sleep disturbance or dizziness and nausea due to orthostatic intolerance, can often be managed effectively.

Difficulties with sleep initiation, sleep phase shift, frequent waking and disturbing nightmares are actively managed with sleep hygiene techniques and melatonin or low dose tricyclic medications such as dothiepin or amitriptyline. Simple migraine prophylactic medications such as pizotifen or periactin are anecdotally effective in reducing the severity of headache. Simple measures such as increasing salt and fluid intake, including electrolyte drinks, and encouraging lower limb exercises and gentle exercise can assist with orthostatic intolerance. Similarly, muscle pain and fibromyalgia can be helped by reducing sleep disturbance and encouraging gentle exercise or physical therapy.

Residual difficulties with concentration, recognition of depression, persistent severe dysmenorrhoea associated with exacerbation of CFS symptoms, ongoing nausea, abdominal discomfort or persistent orthostatic symptoms are usually addressed after review and the implementation of the management plan.

2.3.4 Review appointments

A 6-week follow up appointment is usually scheduled for review of their plan and whether the logistics are sustainable. Residual symptoms are checked including whether the symptom management is appropriate. Any further queries from the young person are addressed. Once a decision had been made regarding the schedule for education, appropriate explanation, documentation, advocacy, extra support, special provision or special consideration is provided or requested. A specific education program to ensure maximum possible opportunity to participate is therefore implemented. Sometimes this requires a combination of Distance Education and school attendance for 1–2 subjects, or attendance for a few classes with visiting teacher assistance. If necessary, the minimum requirements are negotiated to ensure the year level is passed so that they can progress with their peers. Additional details regarding educational strategies used by the Visiting Teacher Service have been documented [27]. If adjustments to sport schedules are required, these are provided and coaches and staff are usually very accommodating once they understand the reasons for the requests.

Generally 3-monthly reviews are arranged to assess progress, educational issues, symptom management and review of goals. Young people are seen more frequently if necessary. Occasionally young people are followed up by a local paediatrician.

In addition, parents often need help navigating the difficult adolescent period and uncertainties regarding assisting with the tasks of adolescent development in the context a chronic illness that is generally not well understood. The developmental tasks (19) of adolescence may fail to progress during the illness and may need to be addressed during management, or time allowed for some catch up when the young person is well enough. Such tasks can be difficult for any parent to navigate but even more difficult when the young person is clearly unwell and not able to manage some simple activities of daily living.

These tasks include increasing sense of independence and responsibility for their actions, peer relationships, sexual identity and development, assessment of risk, sense of self-worth and hope for the future. Persistent dependence, uncertainty about what is required, social anxiety and withdrawal, extreme caution in making decisions, poor self-esteem and depression regarding the future can be the consequence of the limitations imposed by chronic illness. Parents are not sure if they should be defending, protecting and trusting the young person's judgement or cajoling, setting limits and allowing the young person to make mistakes. Many parents put their life 'on hold' to care for the young person with the attendant complications for the whole family, and this often adds significant stressors. For many young people, doing some small chores that do not require much effort is important in order to be part of the family and reduce tensions with siblings.

For younger patients, there are concerns regarding persistent dependence on parents, and anxiety regarding the illness, such as concerns about what was actually wrong and whether there would be recovery. They worry about managing at school, as well as social anxiety when they are absent from their social network for some time. There may also be depression and a sense of helplessness and powerlessness, especially if some family members, the medical profession or teachers do not understand. In addition, the transition into adolescence and secondary school is exacerbated when they are not able to attend frequently enough to engage socially.

2.4 Feedback from young people

Feedback from young people regarding their management was sought on many occasions over the years and has been reported in detail [28]. This feedback modified management. Feedback affirmed that being believed by the clinician, family and school staff and feeling as if they had an advocate to help them navigate the education system were central to their overall ability to cope and their general wellbeing. Having a management framework within which they could organise their priorities was seen as key to feeling as if they could have some control over their life again. Of note, assistance with being able to continue with education was valued as important as their medical management. Continuing social engagement as part of their self-management was crucial for continuing social learning. For those where outpatient support has not been sufficient, there is now access to a 4-week intensive self-management program.

3. The intensive self-management program

3.1 Background

In 2012, the Victorian Paediatric Rehabilitation Service (VPRS) at the RCH in Melbourne commenced multidisciplinary management of adolescents with CFS. This followed a state government review of services available for young people with CFS, and the recognition that outpatient services required additional support and a more coordinated approach. A systematic review by Knight et al. [29], of the limited literature available on paediatric interventions, indicated some support for cognitive behaviour therapy (CBT) and limited support for multidisciplinary intervention. However, the quality of these studies, did not allow firm conclusions to be drawn.

Thus it was decided that the new program would have a CBT framework, be goal-focused and strongly encourage self-management. Following ongoing evaluation and feedback, it was noted that some aspects continued to work well, while others needed modification. With the implication that there is no known 'cure', there needed to be a change in approach from the typical rehabilitation aim of assisting with the reduction of suffering as the sole focus. Feedback from families and participants found this approach to be disempowering. This ensured that, rather than being viewed as an illness to be endured it could be a more hopeful, dynamic and positive process. Recovery was possible and at the very least, there could be an improvement in functioning and some participation in important stages of adolescent development.

In the early years of the program, there was minimal involvement of families in program sessions, with the focus solely on the young person and engaging them in self-management. There was some inflexibility and a more rigid approach where all participants were encouraged to engage in activity on non-program days with little individualization of the program. Often participants were too exhausted at the end of relatively long therapy days to convey to parents what they were keen to practise and how they needed to be supported at home. This resulted in confusion within families about plans and expectations on non-program days, repetition of the same information to multiple people and reduced understanding by parents of the clinical reasoning behind the program. This was an unfortunate approach and much was learnt from patients and families at this time. More flexible, individualised guidance in setting up a management plan was preferred. It allowed for flexibility, review and adjustment when progress occurred. It was noted that family involvement was required to improve participant engagement and successful carryover of effects after the program.

In addition, increasing recognition of the association of postural orthostatic tachycardia syndrome (POTS) in the referrals required a change in the focus of exercise therapy within the program. Cardiologists became an important part of the medical management alongside the CFS medical team.

3.2 Overview of the current 4-week intensive self-management program at RCH

The aim is to encourage ongoing, self-directed learning and management of the illness, so that participants and families have the strategies and confidence to reduce the chaos, uncertainty and loss that underpins living with CFS during adolescence. They are encouraged to re-engage in key areas of life that have been neglected or problematic.

The VPRS CFS Self-Management Program runs for 3 days per week, for a 4-week period and is located in an outpatient setting within the hospital. Four staff, an occupational therapist, a physiotherapist, an education consultant and a clinical psychologist provide interdisciplinary care. Each therapist covers 2 days of the 3-day program. They also meet weekly with referring doctors to discuss participant progress.

A typical day is runs from 9.30 am to 3 pm. Each participant identifies his or her own goals and these are used to establish a framework to work within over the 4 weeks. They continue to work with this framework after the program.

The program is structured around individual and group sessions. The structure of the sessions allows for key content to be explored and built on over the weeks. During the non-program days (two weekdays and the weekend) they are encouraged to practise and to implement what they have learned. Participants are encouraged to be open-minded and to consider new ways of looking at and living their life.

For many participants and families it is an enormous undertaking to attend the program. It varies how feasible it is to practise new skills on non-program days. For most, the opportunity to try out new activities and routines in a considered, modified way is attainable. For some, however, the goal is to engage during program days, learn the theory and skills within the three-day structure and have quiet days in between. Much of the practising then occurs post-program when they can spread their energy availability over a week at a less intense pace. This approach is flexible, individualised and sustainable as they learn self-management tools that continue well beyond the four-week program.

3.3 Assessment

3.3.1 Inclusion criteria

Participant inclusion criteria used by referring doctors from the CFS Outpatient Clinic is as follows:

10–18 years of age.
CFS is the primary diagnosis and the patient accepts this.
Display motivation to engage in the intensive nature of the program.
Enrolment in education.
Physically able to manage 3 days per week of engagement for 4 weeks without significantly worsening their symptoms as a typical program day requires participants to walk approximately 700 m to access the treatment areas from the hospital entrance.
Tried doctor-led outpatient guidance in the first instance.
Stable mental health

This assessment consists of a 45-min psychology assessment, 45-min education assessment and a combined 90-min occupational therapy and physiotherapy assessment. The patient attends the assessment with at least one parent or guardian present. In addition to detailed assessment about CFS, there is exploration of the young person's motivation to participate in a group program setting and their attitudes and beliefs about CFS are recorded. This is to ensure a group program is a suitable 'fit' for the young person. The philosophy and structure of the intervention is explained and goal setting is completed.

We have also noted that if any of the above criteria are not met, the likelihood of positive engagement is poor. In particular, where motivation to participate is parent rather than patient led or if CFS is not the primary diagnosis, the group dynamic is affected.

It is clear that the intensive program is not suitable for all young people with CFS. Those who are unable to attend the program in person for all the required days without significant worsening of symptoms are not appropriate. These patients are encouraged to continue with the doctor-led outpatient guidance in conjunction with a physical therapist that can provide therapy in time frames and intensities that are a better fit for the patient.

Currently the program is moving towards offering pre-program conditioning and guidance to streamline the process of starting a program so that many months are not spent with the young person in limbo.

3.3.2 Baseline and outcome measures

Outcome measures are completed at initial assessment, 6 weeks post-program and 6 months post-program. The current outcome measures are:

- Canadian Occupational Performance Measure (COPM) [30]
- Depression Anxiety Stress Scales (DASS) [31]
- Physical measures—Day 1 sub maximal treadmill test and plank hold
- School attendance

From 2012 to 2018, the psychological measure was the Beck Youth Inventories measure [32].

3.3.3 Assessment decision

The VPRS therapy team meet post-assessment to discuss findings. Provided the patient meets inclusion criteria and the family are keen to participate, an offer is made to participate in an upcoming program. The wait list is usually 2–4 months. If either the family or the VPRS therapists do not feel the 4-week intensive program is an appropriate match for the family, alternatives in the community are explored. We have found that these alternative options are particularly appropriate in cases where families find it too difficult to be at the hospital for the required time due to work, sibling needs or their own health issues.

In addition, as several participants are in each program, every effort is made to match participants based on age, educational stage and likely group dynamic and, to a lesser extent, current function and engagement in life.

3.3.4 Pre-program information and program readiness

Program information is emailed to families soon after an offer is made. This information includes logistics as well as a proposed timetable so that families can forward plan. A blank activity record is also sent to be completed the week prior to the program so that the therapy team have a current record of how the participant is spending each day with regard to sleep, activity, social contact and study.

To give participants the smoothest transition to the program and ultimately an effective intervention, a VPRS therapist via telephone, or in person, conducts a pre-program readiness interview, in the 2 weeks prior to the program. The previously identified program goals are clarified and changed if requested. It has been noted that without adequate time to prepare mentally and physically for the program, it takes longer for participants to settle in and co-operate with the program's agreed expectations.

3.4 Program content

3.4.1 Pacing and energy conservation, sleep, leisure

Participants work as a group to learn and implement core functional activities of daily living into their weekly schedules. Topics covered include sleep hygiene, balancing activity, leisure, memory and concentration, diet, pacing and energy conservation and setback planning. Participants learn to formulate a weekly planner, where they plan a balanced week of both 'need to do' activities and 'want to do' activities. This is to ensure that they plan a manageable week in line with their current baselines of their CFS physical and mental capabilities. During the program, participants embark on an outing as a group in order to practise these concepts and strategies, as also planning and cooking a meal to do the same.

3.4.2 Goal setting

Goal setting sets the framework for the program. Goals are revisited regularly and progress tracked. Weekly individual goal review and progression sessions occur with the Physiotherapist and Occupational Therapist. Weekend planning and weekend review sessions, help to build skills of incorporating structure into to daily routines. These are group sessions and peer feedback is encouraged. In the planning sessions participants generate ideas and suggestions of what is helpful to include in weekends. A key feature of weekend planning is to include leisure activities that the young person has previously enjoyed or is keen to participate in. Weekends are also used for practising independence, perhaps in driving lessons with a parent, taking public transport or helping cook a meal. They are also important opportunities for achieving sleep routine consistency and pacing activity. They also provide an opportunity to practise challenging thoughts and to practise mindfulness and clear communication with family and friends.

3.4.3 Education

Educational engagement is once again identified as the most significant part of life affected by CFS. The effects in a young person's life when school attendance is limited or absent are devastating, affecting self-esteem and mood from social isolation and compromised learning outcomes. Prior to the program the education consultant liaises with participants' school contacts to establish communication. It has been noted that the variability in school engagement prior to the program improves afterwards with schools taking a much greater interest in learning about CFS and how they can assist the young person to engage in school.

During the 4-week program, eight supervised group-learning sessions occur in the Education Institute Learning Space at the hospital where participants undertake private study and complete activities set by their school. They also apply memory and concentration techniques learnt during the program to assist with concentration, pacing, homework and study management. Four individual consultations provide strategies and recommendations for support upon returning to school. These are discussed with the student, family and school personnel. The education consultant continues to support participants and schools well beyond the program to assist with challenges that inevitably arise.

3.4.4 Psychology

The participants receive group psychology sessions weekly wherein they learn the following: (1) understanding how CBT can help; (2) monitoring and challenging thoughts; (3) understanding emotions, stress, anxiety and mood; (4) relaxation strategies for stress and anxiety; (5) coping strategies for low mood; (6) building motivation and (7) engaging in assertive communication skills and family conflict management. In addition to this, they receive individual psychological reviews each week. This builds on the group session work and focuses on assisting with interventions for the interaction between CFS symptoms and mental health.

3.4.5 Physical therapy

The physical therapy component of the program consists of individualised goal setting and program planning based on the initial assessment. It is refined and revised as the program progresses. There is a group theory component as part of some sessions, covering topics such as chronic pain, Postural Orthostatic Tachycardia Syndrome (POTS) and progressing movement and exercise safely in order to minimise the likelihood of post-exertional malaise.

Post-exertional malaise (exhaustion and malaise after activities, either physical or mental, that previously were tolerated well) is a hallmark feature of CFS. It greatly reduces young people's ability to participate in physical activity as previously enjoyed.

Early in the program, participants begin an individualised movement program, delivered in either an individual or small group setting. This starts with gentle stretching and strengthening and for those where it is appropriate, short duration cardio activity. Participants and families are actively involved in all decisions regarding types of reconditioning and pathways of progression.

Participants are given a choice of a range of approaches to movement and reconditioning. They are encouraged to choose activities they have previously enjoyed and would like to incorporate such as shooting goals in basketball outside for a set time with another participant, or completing movements on the pilates reformer machine. Movement tasks are incorporated into weekly plans and are aimed at being meaningful in the young person's life such as walking 5 min to the local shops to buy ingredients to bake or taking the family pet for a walk around the block. Some participants much prefer this approach while others are more aligned with an athlete rehabilitation approach with more conventional exercise. Careful consideration and monitoring is applied to all patients.

3.4.6 Postural Orthostatic Tachycardia Syndrome (POTS)

In recent years, a high number of participants have a diagnosis of POTS alongside CFS. These patients need very specific management in physical therapy sessions. POTS symptoms come on with standing and are relieved when becoming supine. Heart rate increases by 40 beats per minute or more and there can be a blood pressure change. Associated autonomic symptoms include sweating and blueness/swelling in the feet. There are often palpitations, fatigue, exercise intolerance, nausea, near syncope, syncope, 'brain fog' and chronic pain. Doctors may prescribe medications and the exercise component of treatment is critical.

The physical therapy for these patients has four components:

a. **Lower limb and core strengthening.** Lower limb muscles act as a secondary pump to augment venous return. Those patients who are significantly symptomatic start in a reclined sitting position or even in supine position to strengthen all large muscle groups. Exercise therabands are often used for resistance. As symptoms improve, strengthening is completed in standing and progressed with increasing the number of repetitions and resistance.

b. **Cardiovascular reconditioning.** For the most debilitated patients cardiovascular reconditioning starts in a reclined position, usually with pedalling a light set of pedals. The progression is to sit more upright with feet out in front on the pedals and then on to a recumbent exercise bike followed by an upright exercise bike as able. Patients do walk short distances for functional purposes but most of the reconditioning is done in sitting position to reduce the orthostatic load. Sessions are initially short duration and low intensity before progressing in both these areas. Intensity is increased slowly with short duration interval work. Significant consideration and respect is given to fatigue levels and recovery rates.

c. **Standing tolerance drills.** While lower limb and core strengthening and cardiovascular conditioning are developed, some time is devoted, when tolerated, it to starting some exercises in standing position. These include heel raises; squats and wall push ups to challenge the body's ability to exercise while standing.

d. **Additional management.** This includes electrolyte drinks, salt tablets, the wearing of lower body compression garments, raising the bed 10° with the head end higher, and encouraging sitting up with feet flat on the ground rather than lying down during the day. Many patients require medication support to enable the patient to be able to tolerate re-conditioning exercise. When patients present with a POTS diagnosis or have significant orthostatic symptoms, the approach outlined above has been effective. Progression does, however, require a multimodal approach with multidisciplinary input helpful to achieving progress.

Psychology support in POTS patients appears to be very helpful, in particular assisting patients coping with the significant heart rate increases and adrenaline released on upright standing. These physical symptoms mimicking anxiety can be confusing for patients, particularly those where anxiety has not previously been present.

3.4.7 Pain

Pain is a common symptom in CFS. This can be headaches, joint pain or abdominal pain. Very often these pains do not respond to medication. Sometimes pain is present due to long periods of physical inactivity. For other patients the protective function of pain is no longer serving that purpose and patients may develop a central sensitisation.

The approach taken in the program in the first instance is to ascertain a patient's concept of pain. Once this has been established, using questioning and simple quizzes, a pain curriculum is developed. While some initial pain theory is covered in the group setting, further exploration of possible contributing factors to the young person's pain is explored on an individual basis in both physiotherapy and clinical psychology sessions. The treatment approach is based on the work of Lorimer Moseley and David Butler of the Neuro Orthopaedic Institute Australasia [33]. Its focus is on understanding chronic pain as one of many outputs of the brain in response to a range of inputs. It seeks to establish the interactions between the mind, the body and the environment and the complex interaction with the nervous system that occurs.

3.5 Follow-up

Patients are reviewed at 6 weeks and 6 months post-program. There is weekly email or telephone contact in the first 6 weeks post-program with a face-to-face review at 6 weeks. Patients and families are able to access ongoing support from the team for advice and direction. There is limited scope to offer therapist face to face sessions beyond the program outside of the scheduled reviews. All patients return to the care of their referring paediatrician post-program.

3.6 Patient feedback

Feedback is regularly sought from participants—both informally during the program and at follow-up reviews as well as written. More formal feedback has been obtained intermittently. While patients describe learning about pacing, thought challenging and educational tips as being helpful, they overwhelmingly describe meeting other young people in a similar position and feeling like they belong and are supported, as being the most valued part of the program. This often results in participants forming close bonds with each other and many friendships have continued over the years.

4. Review of referrals

As the program is resource intense, and many young people are successfully managed in outpatients, it has been important to attempt to identify which ones need the more concentrated input and access to the multidisciplinary team and when the ideal time is to refer. Approximately 25 complete the program each year. It has been noted that the proportion of males (26%) to females referred to the program reflects the proportion noted over many years of close to 1:3 [10, 15]. However, there was a higher proportion than expected from rural areas. In Victoria, 23% of the population live in the non-metropolitan area, but 42% of participants came from non-metropolitan areas (chi-square 9.19, $p < 0.005$). Rural regions have less access to local paediatricians, additional educational services such as visiting teachers and specialised allied health support is scarce. There were higher proportions of young people participating in the program during year 9 (28%) and year 11 (24%) compared with the other years between grade 6 and year 12. The year 11 students are in their penultimate year of school prior to university entrance exams and year 9 is recognised as a turbulent year in adolescent social development, and the year after which some decisions on subject choices for future careers need to be made. Hence educational issues were a significant stimulus for the referral.

Of note, 44% admitted to >4 h of screen time (phone, computer, television) per day. This would generally be considered excessive but did reflect those who had been unable to increase their school attendance and who had become more socially isolated. It did also become an increasing problem when gaming was involved as this tended to occur late at night and contribute to day/night reversal of sleep cycle and increasing loss of time from school. A higher proportion of males than females saw this as their only social outlet.

POTS was diagnosed in 78% [1, 15] either coinciding with the onset of CFS following an infection, occurring associated with hyperflexibility and having associated CFS symptoms, or apparently developing after the prolonged bed rest or limited activity associated with their CFS. During recent years this has become better recognised, documented and managed but its management has occupied an increasing proportion of referrals. It has generally been poorly recognised by paediatricians and many allied health providers are unfamiliar with how to help especially in the context of the limited stamina of CFS.

From outpatients, it was noted that early referrals to the program were often not appropriate. Young people and their families needed time to understand the illness, develop some confidence that they could plan an appropriate schedule and sustain it, and have an opportunity to improve some of the more troublesome symptoms, such as sleep disturbance and headache. Frequently simple measures for managing POTS or if these were not sufficient, referral to an appropriate cardiologist was important to improve control. Crucially, having a sustainable school program with understanding from school staff and their peers was central to management. Families also needed time to adjust their schedules to a more balanced and sustainable form to assist the young person.

Hence, those who, although they were attending school, struggled with their weekly schedule and balancing their daily activities such as exercise, sleep, school work and social activities needed additional help. Occasionally the family social circumstances made it difficult to attend school regularly. Teachers who were unsympathetic or peers who did not understand contributed to difficulties at school.

Those who were not attending or managing school work, were often very anxious and increasing screen time contributed to further reduction in school attendance. Many found adjusting to avoiding a boom/bust cycle where they would do too much and then take a long time to recover and be very despondent or angry at these restrictions was a significant problem. They felt they needed more support in planning and adapting.

Only a small proportion of the patients seen in the outpatient clinic are referred to the program. As per the feedback over many years, ability to construct a self-management program and guidance to adapt and sustain progress was highly valued. In addition, assistance with planning sustainable education with school liaison was cited as helpful in allowing them to remain socially engaged and hope that their aspirations were achievable. In essence those referred and reporting benefit from the program where those who needed more support in planning their self-management, more intensive assistance for their POTS but most importantly assistance with their education.

It is clear that as the staff have become more familiar with the illness, and have received feedback that they have incorporated into the program, that the key features that are valued are identical to the feedback the outpatient program has received over the years [10, 28]. Access to physiotherapy especially for the specific management of POTS would make outpatient management easier. An education consultant to liaise with schools is often more acceptable for the school than being approached by a paediatrician, although usually medical documentation and recommendations are required by educational authorities. In addition, the input from a psychologist who has an understanding of the illness and the feelings of anxiety that occurs with POTS as well as the impact chronic illness and disrupted education has on the social and emotional development of a young person can be very helpful. Crucially it is the feeling that they are understood and believed and that they are not the only ones with the illness. Regaining some control over their lives by how they can manage the illness is highly valued.

5. Conclusion

The majority of young people can be managed in an outpatient setting and availability of some of the expertise such as physiotherapy and an educational consultant would greatly assist in management in that setting. This would then free the more intensive self-management program for young people who could not access allied health, needed more guidance for planning or who needed help for family understanding, cooperation with school or help to understand the mental health issues that may accompany chronic illness and social isolation. The acceptance and linking with other young people with an illness that is poorly understood and accepted, has been invaluable.

The program at RCH will continue in its current form of individualised patient plans within a group setting. Involvement of families in key sessions alongside participants has shown to be the most effective way to encourage carryover of improved engagement in life post-program.

Ongoing feedback from young people and their families as well as research findings continue to inform both the outpatient management and the intensive VPRS program. Increasing interest and understanding from paediatricians and allied health staff can only help by reducing the frustration, delay, misunderstanding and access to services for these young people. Assisting them with symptom management, guidance in devising and implementing a self-management plan and assistance in navigating the education system has reportedly been highly valued. Having the added assistance of a multidisciplinary team and intensive program when aspects of this management were not sufficient has been highly valued.

Acknowledgements

The frank feedback from the young people regarding their management has been greatly appreciated. The input and support from the team members in the VPRS and the support of A/Prof Adam Scheinberg in setting up and maintaining the program is gratefully acknowledged. There was no external funding for this report.

Conflict of interest

The authors declare no conflict of interest.

Author details

Katherine Rowe[1*], Amanda Apple[2] and Fiona McDonald[1]

1 Department of General Medicine, Royal Children's Hospital, Melbourne, Australia

2 Victorian Paediatric Rehabilitation Service, Royal Children's Hospital, Melbourne, Australia

*Address all correspondence to: kathy@roweresearch.com

References

[1] Rowe PC. Orthostatic intolerance and chronic fatigue syndrome: New light on an old problem. Journal of Pediatrics. 2002;**140**(4):387-389

[2] Holmes GP, Kaplan JE, Gantz NM, et al. Chronic fatigue syndrome: A working case definition. Annals of Internal Medicine. 1988;**108**:387-389

[3] Fukuda K, Strauss S, Hickie I, et al. The chronic fatigue syndrome: A comprehensive approach to its definition and study. Annals of Internal Medicine. 1994;**121**:953-959

[4] Carruthers BM, van de Sande MI, De Meirleir KL, Klimas N, Broderick GG, et al. Myalgic Encephalomyelitis: International Consensus Criteria. 2011. DOI: 10.1111/j.1365-2796.2011.02428.x

[5] Institute of Medicine; Committee on the Diagnostic Criteria for Myalgic Encephalomyelitis/Chronic Fatigue Syndrome. Beyond Myalgic Encephalomyelitis/Chronic Fatigue Syndrome: Redefining an Illness. Washington, DC: The National Academies Press; 2015. DOI: 10.17226/19012

[6] Jason LA, Bell DS, Rowe K, Van Hoof ELS, Jordan KR, Lapp C, et al. A pediatric case definition for myalgic encephalomyelitis and chronic fatigue syndrome. Journal of Chronic Fatigue Syndrome. 2006;**13**:1-44. DOI: 10.1300/J092v13n02_01

[7] Jason LA, Barker A, Brown A. Pediatric myalgic encephalomyelitis/chronic fatigue syndrome. Reviews in Health Care. 2012;**3**(4):257-270

[8] Rowe KS, Rowe KJ. Symptom patterns of children and adolescents with chronic fatigue syndrome. In: Singh NN, Ollendick TH, Singh AN, editors. International Perspectives on Child and Adolescent Mental Health. Vol. 2. New York: Elsevier Science; 2002. pp. 395-415

[9] Rowe KS, Rowe KJ. Symptom patterns and psychological features of adolescents with chronic fatigue syndrome. Journal of Paediatrics & Child Health. 2005;**41**(8):S9 August [Paediatrics and Child Health Division The Royal Australasian College of Physicians: Paediatric Abstracts presented at the Annual Scientific Meeting, May 2005: Paediatrics & Child Health Divisional Abstracts and Posters: 2005]

[10] Rowe KS. Long term follow up of young people with chronic fatigue syndrome attending a pediatric outpatient service. Frontiers in Pediatrics. 2019;7:21. DOI: 10.3389/fped.2019.00021

[11] Friedman KJ. Advances in ME/CFS: Past, present, and future. Frontiers in Pediatrics. 2019. DOI: 10.3389/fped.2019.00131

[12] Bell DS, Jordan K, Robinson M. Thirteen-year follow-up of children and adolescents with chronic fatigue syndrome. Pediatrics. 2001;**107**(5):994-998

[13] Rowe KS. 5-year follow-up of young people with chronic fatigue syndrome following the double-blind randomised controlled intravenous gammaglobulin trial. Journal of Chronic Fatigue Syndrome. 1999;**5**(3/4):97-107

[14] Rowe KS. Chronic fatigue syndrome. In: Kang M, Skinner SR, Sanci LA, Sawyer SM, editors. Youth Health and Adolescent Medicine. East Hawthorn, Vic: IP Communications; 2013. pp. 343-360

[15] Rowe PC, Underhill RA, Friedman KJ, Gurwitt A, Medow MS, Schwartz MS, et al. Myalgic encephalomyelitis/chronic

fatigue syndrome diagnosis and management in young people: A primer. Frontiers in Pediatrics. 2017;**5**:121. DOI: 10.3389/fped.2017.00121

[16] Crawley E, Sterne JA. Association between school absence and physical function in paediatric chronic fatigue syndrome/myalgic encephalopathy. Archives of Disease in Childhood. 2009;**94**:752-756. DOI: 10.1136/adc.2008.143537

[17] Crawley EM, Emond AM, Sterne JAC. Unidentified chronic fatigue syndrome/myalgic encephalomyelitis (CFS/ME) is a major cause of school absence: Surveillance outcomes from school-based clinics. BMJ Open 2011;**1**:e000252. DOI: 10.1136/bmjopen-2011-000252

[18] Knight SJ, Politis J, Garnham C, Scheinberg A, Tollit MA. School functioning in adolescents with chronic fatigue syndrome. Frontiers in Pediatrics. 2018. DOI: 10.3389/fped.2018.00302

[19] Suris J-C, Michaud P-A, Viner R. The adolescent with a chronic condition. Part I: Developmental issues. Archives of Disease in Childhood. 2004;**89**:938-942. DOI: 10.1136/adc.2003.045369

[20] Holmes AM, Deb P. The effect of chronic illness on the psychological health of family members. The Journal of Mental Health Policy and Economics. 2003;**6**(1):13-22

[21] Lloyd AR, Wakefield D, Boughton C, Dwyer J. What is myalgic encephalomyelitis? Lancet. 1988;**1**(8597):1286-1287

[22] Rowe KS. Double blind placebo controlled trial to assess the efficacy of intravenous gammaglobulin for the management of chronic fatigue syndrome in adolescents. Journal of Psychiatric Research. 1997;**31**(1):133-147

[23] Lloyd A, Hickie I, Wakefield D, Boughton C, Dwyer J. A double-blind placebo-controlled trial of intravenous immunoglobulin therapy in patients with the chronic fatigue syndrome. The American Journal of Medicine. 1990;**89**:561-568

[24] Peterson PK, Shepard J, Macres M, et al. A controlled trial of intravenous immunoglobulin G in chronic fatigue syndrome. The American Journal of Medicine. 1990;**89**:554-560

[25] Vollmer-Conna U, Hickie I, Hadzi-Pavlovic D, Tymms K, Wakefield D, Dwyer J, et al. Intravenous immunoglobulin is ineffective in the treatment of patients with chronic fatigue syndrome. The American Journal of Medicine. 1997;**103**(1):38-43

[26] Goldenring JM, Cohen E. H.E.A.D.S.S.—Getting into adolescent heads. Contemporary Pediatrics. 1998;**5**:75-90

[27] Rowe KS, Fitzgerald P. Educational strategies for chronically ill students: Chronic fatigue syndrome. The Australian Educational and Developmental Psychologist. 1999;**16**(2):5-21

[28] Rowe KS. Paediatric patients with myalgic encephalomyelitis/chronic fatigue syndrome value understanding and help to move on with their lives. Acta Paediatr. 18 December 2019. DOI: 10.1111/apa.15054. [Epub ahead of print]

[29] Knight SJ, Scheinberg A, Harvey AR. Interventions in pediatric chronic fatigue syndrome/myalgic encephalomyelitis: A systematic review. Journal of Adolescent Health. 2013;**53**(2):154-165. DOI: 10.1016/j.jadohealth.2013.03.009

[30] Law M, Baptiste S, McColl M, Opzoomer A, Polatajko H, Pollock N. The Canadian occupational performance measure: An outcome measure for occupational therapy. Canadian Journal

of Occupational Therapy. 1990;**57**(2): 82-87. DOI: 10.1177/000841749005700207

[31] Lovibond SH, Lovibond PF. Manual for the Depression Anxiety Stress Scales. Sydney, NSW: The Psychology Foundation of Australia; 1995

[32] Beck JS, Beck AT, Jolly JB. Beck Youth Inventories—Second Edition (BYI–2). Toronto, Ontario: Psychology Corporation; 2005

[33] Butler DS, Moseley GL. Explain Pain: (Revised and Updated). 2nd ed. Adelaide: Noigroup Publications; 2013

Chapter 2

Minor Surgery in Primary Care

Jose Maria Arribas Blanco, Wafa Elgeadi Saleh, Belén Chavero Méndez and María Alvargonzalez Arrancudiaga

Abstract

Minor surgical procedures are defined as a set of procedures in which short surgical techniques are applied on superficial tissues, usually with local anesthesia, and minimal complications, that usually do not require postoperative resuscitation and need minimal equipment, many of which are used on a daily basis, and can be easily and safely performed in a short amount of time during clinic visit. General practitioners should have an optimal infrastructure and medical furniture in a minor surgery operating room. It is important to manage the instruments and materials involved for basic and advanced surgery. Also, for a good clinical practice in minor surgery, it is necessary that general practitioners handle anesthesia techniques (local anesthetic infiltration and regional blocks) and have knowledge of the body areas of risk in minor surgery and the topographic anatomy of the skin for the right performance of surgical procedure. The patients should be informed about the procedure and its technical details before asking them to sign the informed consent form.

Keywords: ambulatory surgical procedures, sutures, minor surgical procedures, electrocoagulation, anesthetics, local, lipoma, keratosis, actinic

1. Introduction

This chapter will try and help general practitioners master minor surgical procedures.

General practitioners require these procedures for diagnostic or therapeutical reasons, in the outpatient setting as well in the emergency (excision of skin lesions or wound suturing for example). For that reason, the training of the general doctors in minor surgery is an additional tool for good medical practice and acquiring skills in minor surgical procedures has become a critical part of medical training.

Minor surgical procedures do not involve very sophisticated devices. However, some basic requirements in terms of infrastructure and equipment must be met [1, 2].

It is recommended that each facility has a specific room for these procedures. This room (**Figure 1**) must include:

Surgical room: a well-ventilated room, with a suitable temperature, it is imperative that is clean, but it does not require sterile isolation. The surgical room should be cleaned properly at the end of the surgical session, particularly after contaminated procedures (e.g. abscesses).

Operating table: It should be easily accessible from all sides, Height-adjustable and articulated tables. It is essential that allows the doctor to work in comfort, both standing and sitting.

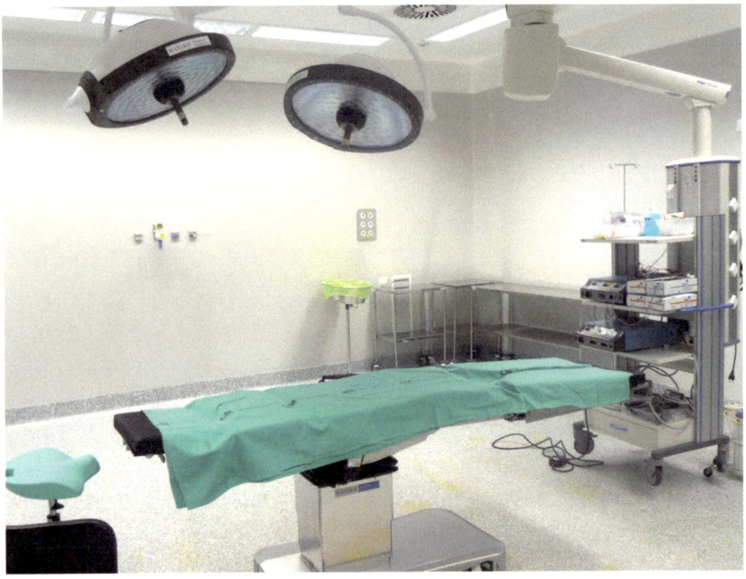

Figure 1.
Well-equipped room of minor surgery.

Doctor's stool: A height-adjustable stool on wheels.

Side table: it is used to place the surgical instruments and material used during the surgery.

Lamp: It is necessary to have a directional light source, and it must provide adequate lighting with, at least, 45,000 lux of illuminance. It is advisable to have another auxiliary lamp with a magnifying glass.

Showcase and containers: For storing consumables and surgical instruments. There should also be properly marked containers for bio contaminated material, and a disposal system in accordance with current health legislation.

Resuscitation equipment: Including material for vascular access, airway intubation, saline, drugs for resuscitation (e.g. epinephrine, atropine, bicarbonate) and a defibrillator.

2. Sterilization system

2.1 Physician's preparation for minor surgery

Performing minor surgical procedures carries some risk of transmission of infectious diseases (such as HCV and HIV), both from patient to doctor and vice versa. To minimize this risk, all physicians performing invasive procedures should adopt and apply universal precautions, which include:

Surgical attire: surgical shirts and trousers ("scrubs") or gowns and sterile gloves. Surgical masks and eye goggles is considered highly desirable but not essential. Disposable gowns are very useful.

Hand washing: Hygienic scrubbing is suitable for minor surgery and involves using a normal soap solution (no brush) and washing thoroughly all skin folds for at least 20 seconds. Time span from scrubbing to glove placement should never exceed 10 minutes.

Sterile glove placement: Outer surface of the glove should be sterile, therefore they cannot be touched with the hands, only with the other glove; nonetheless, the inner or powdered part of the glove can be touched.

3. Surgical instruments (handling) and suture material

3.1 Surgical instruments for minor surgery

The quality, condition and type of instruments used in any procedure can affect its outcome. Choosing the right instruments for each surgical intervention is, therefore, an important issue [1].

Scalpel: A number 3 handle with leaves number 15 for dissection and 11 for incisions and withdrawal of points. The scalpel blade is installed on the handle in a unique position, matching the blade guide with the handle guide. The scalpel is handled with the dominant hand like a pencil (**Figure 2**), allowing small and precise incisions. To increase precision, hand should be partially supported on the working surface. Skin should be tightened perpendicularly to the direction of the incision using the contralateral hand, cutting the skin perpendicularly. In hairy areas (eyebrows or scalp), to avoid damaging the follicles, the incision should be parallel to the hairshafts.

Scissors: The scissors allows us both the cutting dissection of the tissues and the blunt dissection.

A 14 cm long curved blunt May scissors (cutting scissors) and an 11.5 cm curved blunt Metzenbaum scissors (dissecting scissors) should be available.

Scissors are handled by inserting the distal phalange of the thumb and fourth finger into the rings, then supporting the second finger on the branches of the scissors. Usually scissors are inserted with the tip closed and are then opened, separating the tissues in the anatomical layers, except for sharp dissection they are inserted with the tip open, then cutting the tissue.

Needle-holder: needle-holders are meant to hold curved needles while stitching. The needle is held 2/3 of the way back from its point. A small or medium (12–15 cm). Long needle holders are not recommended.

Like other instruments with rings, the needle support is handled equally. To facilitate the passage of the needle through the tissues, the needle holder should describe a prono-supination movement, and for a proper edge eversion of the wound the angle of entry of the needle should be 90°. The non-dominant hand holds the skin with a retractor or dissecting forceps, opposing the pressure of the needle.

Dissecting forceps: Use of a 12 cm-long Adson forceps with teeth to handle the skin, plus a toothless Adson forceps for suture removal or two standard forceps, one with and one without teeth. It is important not to manipulate the skin using non-toothed forceps.

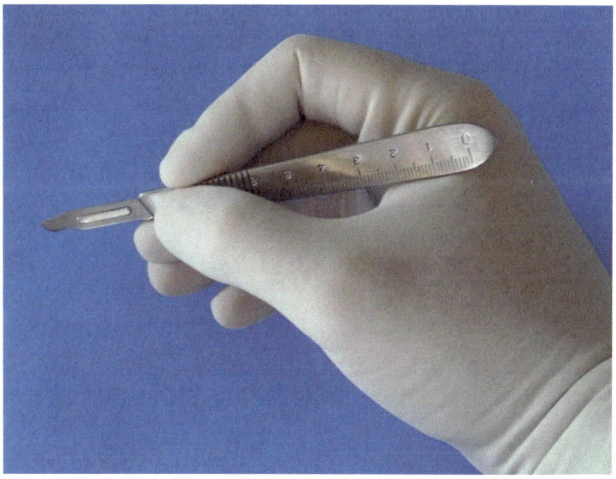

Figure 2.
Correct way of managing of the scalpel.

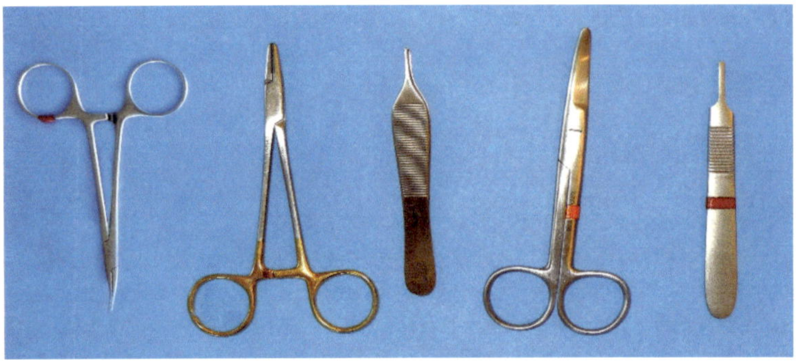

Figure 3.
Basic set of instruments of minor surgery: Scalpel (handle of the number 3 for scalpel number 15), scissors of May, Adson forceps with teeth, needle-holders and mosquito forceps.

They used with the non dominant hand, between the first, second and third fingers. They allow the surgeon to expose the tissues to manipulate them.

Homeostats: homeostats are used to pull tissue, for homeostasis and, in some cases, for blunt dissection in absence of small scissors. Usually with 12 cm curved non-toothed Mosquito forceps.

For most minor surgical interventions, a basic set of surgical instruments is enough (**Figure 3**). But some surgical procedures require the use of special instruments or equipment, such as:

Biopsy punch: it is an instrument consisting of a handle and a cylindrical cutting edge (trephine) for obtaining tissue biopsies. It allows the surgeon to obtain full-thickness samples of the skin.

The most useful in minor surgery is the 4 mm punch but they are manufactured in different diameters. They are handled with the dominant hand, performing rotational movements of the instrument to cut the skin and obtain the sample [3].

Curette: it allows scraping of lesions on the skin Surface with a simple surgical technique that involves "scraping" or enucleating different types of superficial, hyperkeratotic or raised partial-thickness skin lesions.

Cryosurgical equipment: these are devices that spray a cryogen, which is usually liquid nitrogen that uses extremely cold temperatures to treat benign and malignant skin lesions (solar lentigines, common warts, myxoid cysts, actinic keratosis, etc.).

It is available, cost-effective, and rapid treatment that rarely requires anesthesia [4].

Electrocautery: it applies an electric current with ability to coagulate and cut through different tissues. There are different terminals depending on the type of procedure that is to be performed [5].

3.2 Suture materials

Different types of suture materials are available: threads, staples, adhesive sutures and tissue adhesives.

Depending on the material used for the suture, the operation time will be modified and will require anesthesia or not.

Conventional sutures require the use of anesthesia, operating time is increased, and tissue is traumatized, but provide a secure wound closure and minimal wound-dehiscence rate compared to other types of closure [6].

3.2.1 Sutures

They are classified according to their origin (natural, such as silk, or synthetic polymers that produce less tissue reaction), their configuration (monofilament or

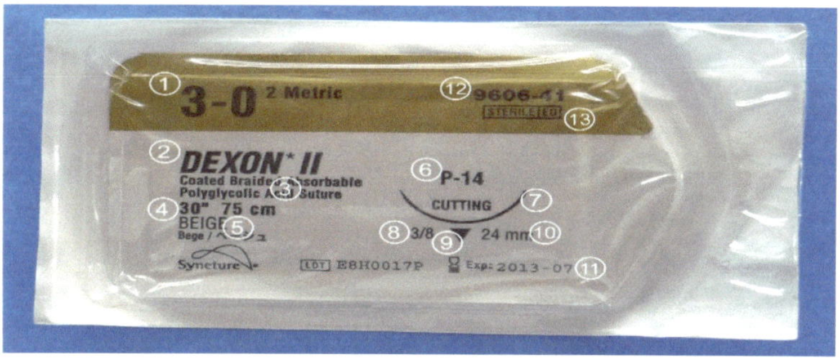

Figure 4.
Information on suture: (1) caliber of the thread (system USP and metric), (2) trade name of the suture, (3) composition and physical structure of the thread, (4) length of the thread, (5) color of the thread, (6) model of needle (every manufacturer uses different references), (7) I draw from the needle to scale 1:1, (8) circumference of the needle (expressed in parts of circle), (9) section of the needle, (10) length of the needle, (11) expiry date, (12) indexes of the manufacturer, (13) indicator of sterile packing.

multifilament), and their size (the thickness of the suture is measured using a zero-scale [USP system] (**Figure 4**). The most commonly used in minor surgery range from 2/0 to 4/0 or 5/0.

The size and type of suture will be selected depending on the anatomical site, the type of wound and on the patient's features.

3.2.1.1 Features of main sutures

- *Nonabsorbable sutures*: They are not degraded by the body and they are used for skin wounds in which stitches that are to be removed or for internal structures that must maintain a constant tension (like tendons and ligaments), Polypropylene and Nylon, causes minimal tissue reaction.

    1. Silk: Suitable for skin suture and for removable sutures in general, it is easy to handle and tie.

    2. Nylon: Indicated for precise skin sutures and internal structures that must maintain constant tension.

    3. Polypropylene: Indicated in continuous intradermal skin closure. It is a very soft suture with high package memory and, therefore, it requires more knots for secure tying, and it is more expensive than Nylon.

- *Absorbable sutures*: A suture is considered absorbable if, when placed under the skin surface, it loses most of its tensile strength in 60 days. It has low tissue reactivity, high tensile strength. They are use in dermal suturing, subcutaneous tissue, deep suturing and ligatures of small vessels. The most commonly used, are the synthetic sutures (polyglactin 910 [Vicryl], polyglycolic acid [Dexon]...).

3.2.1.2 Stitch removal

The period of time (in days) recommended for the extraction of points, together with an indication of the type of suture is described in **Table 1**.

3.2.2 Suturing needles

Needle selection depends on the type of tissue to be sutured, its accessibility and suture thickness.

Anatomical region	Skin suturing	Subcutaneous suturing (Vicryl® or Dexon®)	Stitch removal	
			Adults	children
Scalp	Staples 2/0 silk	3/0	7–9	6–8
Eyelids	6/0 monofilament or silk	—	3–5	3–5
Ears	4/0–5/0 monofilament or silk	—	4–5	3–5
Face, neck, nose, forehead	4/0 monofilament or silk	4/0	4–6	3–5
Lips	4/0 monofilament or silk	4/0	4–6	4–5
Trunk/abdomen	3/0–4/0 monofilament	3/0	7–12	7–9
Back			12–14	14
Lower extremity	3/0 monofilament	3/0	8–12	7–10
Penis	4/0 monofilament	3/0	7–10	6–8
Foot and pulp of fingers			10–12	8–10
Upper limb/hand			8–10	7–9
Mouth and tongue	3/0 Vicryl®	—	—	—

Table 1.
Indications of types of sutures and time for stitch removal.

Needles are classified as triangular, spatulate or conical, according to their section. Triangular needles are considered the first choice in minor surgery, as they have sharp edges that allow suturing through highly-resistant tissues such as subcutaneous tissue, skin or fascia.

Curved needles are used with the needle holder, that is designed to hold needles atraumatically and safely. Short needle holders are preferred in minor surgery; however, they should be selected in accordance with the size of the needle and the surgical area.

3.2.3 Staples

Staples are applied by disposable staplers and they are available in different widths (R: normal staples, W: Wide staples). Staplers are preloaded with a variable number of staples. It has certain advantages such as the speed with which the suture is performed, low resistance and no tissue reaction.

They are applied with the dominant hand, while the non dominant hand everts the skin edges using dissecting forceps with teeth. Staple removal is performed using a staple extractor.

Indications: In linear wounds on the scalp, trunk and limbs, and for temporary closure of wounds in patients to be transferred or with other serious injuries.

Contraindications: Wounds on face and hands and regions that are going to be studied through CT or MRI.

3.2.4 Adhesive sutures

It consists of adhesive tapes made of porous paper and capable of approximating the edges of a wound or incision. They are available in various widths and lengths, and it can be cut.

Indications: linear and superficial wounds with little tension. The regions where they are used most are: the face, chest, non-articular surfaces of the limbs and fingertips. They are also a good choice for elderly patients and to wound-reinforcement after stitch removal.

Any wound closed with adhesive suture should not be wet for the first few days, due to the risk of tape detachment.

Contraindications: irregular wounds, on the scalp and hairy areas, skin folds and joint surfaces.

Application and removal of adhesive sutures: For a good application the wound should be free of blood or secretions and dry. The suture tape is applied to the wound using dissecting forceps without teeth or fingers, first on one edge of the wound and then the other and along the wound.

Time for adhesive suture removal parallels time for conventional suture.

3.2.5 Tissue adhesives (glues)

These products (cyanoacrylates) act as an adhesive, producing an epidermal plane closure, so they bind the most superficial epithelial layer (stratum corneum) and hold together the wound edges for 7–14 days. After this time, adhesive and stratum corneum are shed along.

Adhesive can be used in deeper wounds or with great tension, associated at sutures in the subcutaneous plane.

It have advantages when compared with sutures: More rapid repair time, less painful procedure, better acceptance by patients, no need for suture removal or follow-up, good cosmetically results. Finally they are safer than sutures because needlesticks are avoided [1, 7].

3.2.5.1 Application technique

After cleanliness and hemostasis of the wound, tissue adhesive will be applied:

- Using fingers or dissecting forceps to approximate the wound edges, apply the adhesive on the outer surface of the skin. Then Keep the edges in contact for 30–60 seconds. The process can be repeated 3 times.

- The wound does not require dressings but should be kept dry 5 days. The glue will disappear after 7–10 days.

3.2.5.2 Warnings for correct use

If adhesive contact the eyes, use of a generous amounts of ophthalmic antibiotic ointment should be placed within the eye and on the eyelid to break down the adhesive and reopening of eyelids with a gentle manual traction. If adhesive reach the cornea, it should be assessed for corneal abrasion.

4. Surgical procedures and techniques of anesthesia in minor surgery

4.1 Basic surgical maneuvers

The practice of any surgical procedure, however minimal, is not without risks. The possibility of complications during and after surgery must always be kept in mind. The results of surgical treatment are not always predictable, and depend on many factors, involving not only the physician's skills, but also the patient.

4.1.1 Surgical incision and dissection

There are two ways to dissect tissue: with a blunt dissection, separating the tissue, using Metzenbaum scissors or mosquito forceps, or cutting dissection, with a scalpel or scissors.

4.1.1.1 Incisions shape in minor surgery

Incisions must parallel the minimal tension lines, which match skin relaxation lines and facial expression. Thus, they result in an acceptable scar, both functionally and cosmetically. There are diagrams of the relaxed skin tension lines, for correct incision planning before surgery.

The incision can be marked prior to skin antiseptic preparation or a previously sterilized marking pen can be used in the surgical field after skin preparation and draping.

For excisional biopsies, it is necessary to leave an adequate margin (1–2 mm) of healthy skin both around the lesion and in depth, depending on each lesion.

4.1.1.2 Types of incisions for minor surgery

Incision: Used for drainage of abscesses or surgical exposure of deeper tissues (e.g., epidermal cysts, lipomas, lymph node biopsies). Depending of surgery or the anatomic area, Incisions can be angled, curved or straight.

Elliptical excision: Its should be oriented along the lines of minimal tension.

Usually the length of the ellipse should be 3 times its width and the ends form a 30° angle. Its used to remove skin lesions with a margin of healthy skin in depth and around lesion, and include all skin layers plus some subcutaneous fat (**Figure 5**). This technique allows diagnosis, treatment and facilitates closure producing good cosmetic results.

It is the ideal technique to remove the majority of skin lesions [8–10].

The procedure involves the following steps:

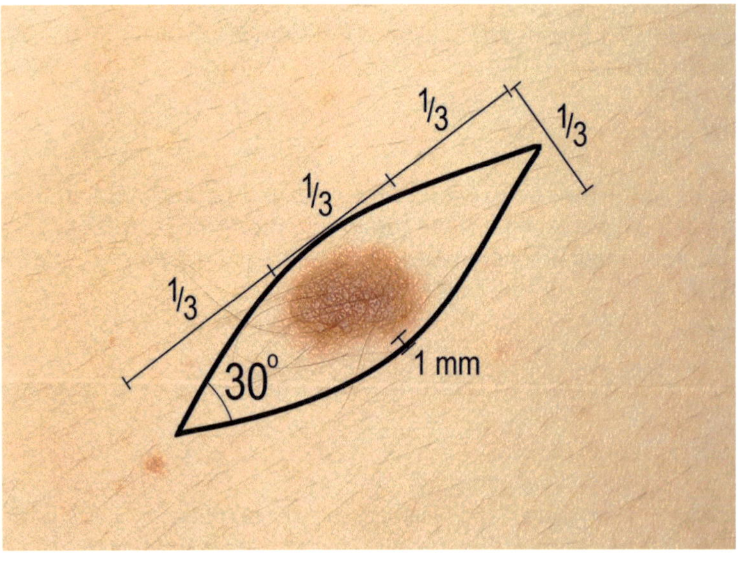

Figure 5.
Characteristics of the elliptical excision.

1. Design of the incision

2. Preparation of the surgical field

3. Local anesthetic injection.

4. Superficial skin incision along the marked ellipse, going through the entire dermis to prevent jagged edges.

5. Using the nondominant hand the deep wedge-shaped incision is made (always under direct vision), until fat is reached and the lesion is, thus, removed en bloc.

6. Hemostasis of the surgical area.

7. Wound closure by layers

8. Cleaning the surgical area and dressing placement

9. After 48 hours the wound can be washed gently

Tangential excision: it is the technique of choice to remove very superficial lesions using scalpel or scissors, eliminating only the most superficial layers of the skin and for which diagnosis is certain. The defect created is allowed to heal by secondary intention. Tangential excision also called "skin shave".

No surgical procedure is complete until the pathology report has been received and the patient informed of the results and prognosis.

4.1.2 Hemostasis

Most episodes of bleeding in minor surgery can be controlled with pressure with a gauze or a surgical towel. It is recommended to apply a compressive bandage on the wound in the immediate postoperative period to reduce hematoma or seroma.

4.1.2.1 Types of hemostasis

Tourniquet: Its allows the exploration of the wound and reduces the surgical time. Its use is limited to distal areas (the fingers nail surgery, etc.) and should not exceed 15 minutes.

- *The hemostats*: The surgeon holds bleeding vessel with the tip of a hemostat without teeth and controls the bleeding. To avoid damaging important structures (for example, tendons or nerves) it is necessary to identify the bleeding vessel.

- *The ligatures*: they are threads that tied around a blood vessel, occlude their light and prevent bleeding. After that, vessel should be fixed with a hemostat. The ligature should pass under the clamp and several knots must be tied.

- In the hemostasis by electrocoagulation, the Bovie is used in coagulation mode.

4.1.3 Suture techniques

4.1.3.1 Interrupted sutures

This is the most appropriate for minor surgery, as it helps to distribute stress, and promotes the drainage of the wound. The number of sutures needed varies according to the length, shape and location of the laceration. In general, the sutures are placed away from each other so that no space appears on the edges of the wound.

Simple stitch (percutaneous): It is used alone or in combination with buried stitches in deeper wounds and it is considered the technique of choice.

Simple stitch with buried knot: Used to reduce tension within the wound and approximate the deep planes, before skin suturing. Absorbable material is used, the knot leaving in the depth of the wound, and is cut flush.

Mattress stitch or "U" stitch: It is useful in areas of loose skin (e.g., elbow, back of the hand), where the wound edges tend to invaginate. In addition this suture provides good obliteration of dead space, avoiding the need for buried sutures in shallow wounds.

- Horizontal mattress stitch: provides a good eversion of wound edges, especially in areas where the dermis is thick or with high tension [6]

- Half-buried horizontal mattress stitch: is used to suture wound angles or surgical edges of uneven thickness.

4.1.3.2 Running sutures

They are contraindicated if an infection is suspected and in very contaminated wounds.

Simple running suture: is a sequence of points with an initial knot and a final knot. It takes a short time to do it, but it makes it difficult to adjust the tension of the skin. It is rarely used in minor surgery.

Continuous intradermal suture (subcuticular): this type of suture allows the wound to be sutured without breaking the skin, avoids the "cross-hatching" and provides an optimal esthetic result. Non-absorbable monofilament suture material or absorbable material can be used. Intradermal sutures are used in wounds where it will be necessary to maintain the suture for more than 15 days. In minor surgery its usefulness is limited.

4.1.3.3 Knot-tying

When a multifilament yarn is knotted (for example, Silk), three loops are usually sufficient (first a double loop plus two simple loops). When knotting a monofilament yarn (e.g., Nylon, polypropylene), an additional loop must be added to increase knot security. The knots should be placed on one side of the wound, rather than placed on top of the incision. This will allow a better visualization of the wound and will interfere less with the healing and facilitate the removal of points.

4.2 Local anesthesia in minor surgery

Local anesthetics block the transmission of nerve impulses and they causing, the absence of sensation in a specific part of the body, also other local senses may be affected.

Local anesthetics can be classified into two groups: esters and amides (lidocaine, mepivacaine, bupivacaine, prilocaine, etidocaine and ropivacaine). For their remarkable safety and efficacy we will only use amides. The association of vasoconstrictors allows better visualization of the surgical field. The most widely used is adrenaline and the maximum dose must not exceed 250 micrograms in adults or 10 micrograms/kg in children [11].

4.2.1 Available presentations

The concentration of the anesthetic is expressed in %. We must know that a concentration of 1% means that 100 ml of the solution contain 1 g of anesthetic. Therefore a 2 ml ampoule of 2% mepivacaine, its contain 40 mg (**Table 2**).

4.2.2 Use of vasoconstrictors

Due to the risk of necrosis and other alteration like delayed healing, adrenaline should not be used in acral areas (e.g., toes), or in traumatized and devitalized skin.

4.2.3 Basic techniques of local anesthesia

4.2.3.1 Topical anesthesia

It is use in an intact skin and for lacerations and mucosae, especially in children. And their characteristics are shown in the **Table 2**.

4.2.3.2 Infiltration anesthesia

1. *Angular infiltration*: From the point of entry, the anesthetic is infiltrated in three or more different directions, like a fan (**Figure 6**).

2. *Perilesional infiltration*: Starting from each point of entry the anesthetic is infiltrated in a single direction. The different points of entry will be forming a polyhedral figure.

Anesthetic	Mode of use	characteristics	Indications	Complications	Not indicated
LET® (4% lidocaine, 0.1% epinephrine 1:2000, 0.5% tetracaine)	1–3 ml applied directly on wound for 15–30 minutes	Onset 20–30 minutes after application.	Can be effective in children for face and scalp lacerations and less effective in limbs	No important adverse effects reported	For mucosae and acral areas
EMLA® lidocaine 25 mg/ml plus prilocaine 25 mg/ml,	1–2 g of cream should be applied for each 10 cm^2 of intact skin and occluded. Maximum dose is 10 g	Onset 60–120 minutes after application. Duration of effect is 30–120 minutes. Not useful on palms of hands and soles of feet	Admitted for procedures on intact skin: scraping and shaving, cryosurgery, electrosurgery, laser hair removal, pre-anesthesia for infiltration	Local mild irritation, contact dermatitis. There have been reports of Methemoglobinemia in children aged <6 months	For wounds or deep tissues

Table 2.
Topical anesthetics used in minor surgical procedures and their characteristics.

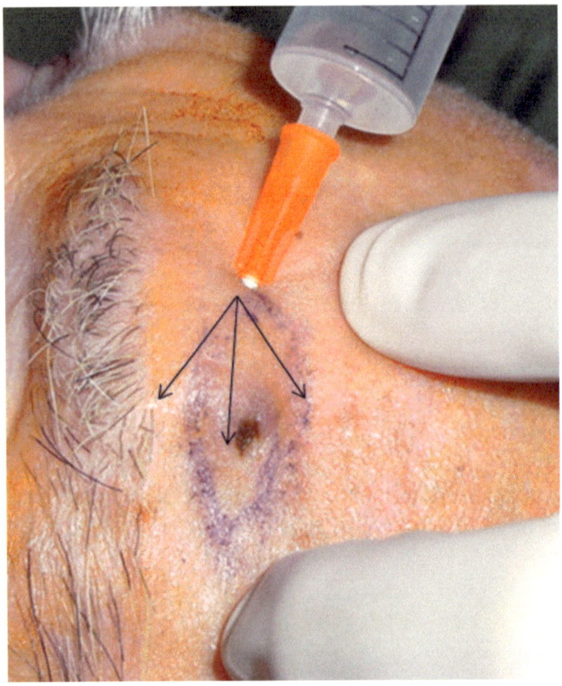

Figure 6.
Anesthetic angular infiltration: it infiltrates following three or more different directions, like a fan.

3. *Linear infiltration*: If the lesion to be operated on is a skin laceration, the anesthetic should be directly infiltrated into the wound edges in a linear fashion. If the wound is bruised and has irregular edges, it is preferable to use a perilesional technique from the uninjured area, and follow along the margins of the wound to avoid introducing microbial contamination.

4.2.3.3 Loco-regional block

The needle is inserted at the base of the proximal phalanx in a dorsal and lateral location, in the collateral palmar digital nerve, and then local anesthetic is injected (maximum 4 ml). The needle is removed and after aspiration proceeds to infiltrate again the subcutaneous plane.

The surgeon must wait 10–15 minutes to obtain a complete effect of the blockage.

5. Preoperative considerations

5.1 Diagnostic criteria for the most common lesions in minor surgery

It is important that general practitioners have an extensive knowledge of the lesions most frequently treated by minor surgery [12].

The following paragraphs contain an overview of the most important diagnostic consideration in lesions usually treated with minor surgery.

5.1.1 Seborrheic keratoses

These lesions are easily treated with curettage, electrosurgery or cryosurgery. In case of doubt, an incisional biopsy should be sent for histopathological analysis.

5.1.2 Epidermal cysts

They are also known as epithelial cysts, epidermoid cysts, or improperly, "sebaceous cysts." The cyst wall consists of normal stratified squamous epithelium derived from the follicular infundibulum. Queratin is the main component inside the cyst. Their treatment is surgical removal for cosmetic reasons or due to recurrent infections.

5.1.3 Warts

They are a form of benign epithelial hyperplasia induced by the human papillomavirus (HPV). Clinical presentations of cutaneous HPV infection include:

Verruca Vulgaris or plantar wart: you can use liquid nitrogen or salicylic acid.

5.1.4 Molluscum

It is presents as pearly white papules of 1–5 mm (sometimes even bigger) with central dimpling. They may appear isolated or in groups in the neck, trunk, anogenital area or eyelids. Their first choice treatment is cryosurgery, curettage.

5.1.5 Lipoma

Lipomas are slow-growing benign tumors of mature adipose tissue. They appear as soft, elastic, smooth or multilobulated tumors of variable size, with ill-defined borders, and not adherent to deep planes. The diagnosis is usually made clinically. But ultrasound can be helpful to distinguish a lipoma from an epidermoid cyst or a ganglion cyst [13]. They are generally asymptomatic and they are treated by surgical removal [2].

5.1.6 Fibroma pendulum, skin tags

They are not malignant and their treatment is justified for cosmetic reasons.

5.1.7 Melanocytic nevi

They are acquired lesions in the form of macules or papules or small nodules (<1 cm) and are constituted by groups of melanocytes located in the epidermis, dermis or both areas and rarely in the subcutaneous tissue. Sun exposure contributes to the induction of these lesions.

5.1.8 Actinic keratosis

It is located in sun-exposed areas such as bald scalp, the face, shoulders, ears, neck and the back of the hands. It is caused by damage from exposure to ultraviolet radiation. Actinic keratoses are more prevalent in males of middle-aged.

Actinic keratosis is considered a precancer. 13–25% it could develop into a squamous cell carcinoma.

If lesions are scarce and localized, they may be treated with liquid nitrogen.

5.1.9 Basal cell carcinoma

It is the most common skin malignancy. Approximately 70% of basal cell carcinoma occurs on the face, and 15% presents on the trunk [14]. Exposure to ultraviolet (UV) radiation in sunlight, especially during childhood, is the most important factors that contribute to the development of Basal cell carcinoma.

5.1.10 Squamous cell carcinoma

This is a malignant tumor that usually appears on a previous premalignant lesion and requires a multidisciplinary therapeutical approach involving dermatologists, surgeons, radiotherapists, and chemotherapists [14].

5.1.11 Melanoma

Of all skin malignancies, melanoma has the worst prognosis, Five-year survival rates for people with melanoma depend on the stage of the disease at the time of diagnosis.

5.2 Body areas of risk in minor surgery

High-risk areas for minor surgery include the facial and cervical regions, axillary and supraclavicular regions, wrists, hands and fingers, the groin, the popliteal fossa and the feet.

We must consider those regions with a greater tendency to develop pathological scars (e.g., shoulder, sternal and interscapular region). Also the skin of black patients and children are especially prone.

6. Good clinical practice in minor surgery

6.1 Preoperative

For most basic minor surgical procedures, no preoperative work-up is needed. **Table 3** summarizes the precautions of minor surgery in primary care.

In patients with increased anxiety, 5–10 mg oral or sublingual diazepam, or 1–5 mg sublingual lorazepam can be administered 30 minutes before surgery.

Contraindications for minor surgery: Malignant skin lesion, allergy to local anesthetics, pregnancy (surgery should be deferred until the end of pregnancy, if malignancy is suspected, the patient should be referred to a specialist), an acute illness, doubt about patient's motivations, patients with psychiatric disorders or

-Surgery in the lower extremities in patients with Diabetes Mellitus and peripheral vascular disease. -In patients with arrhythmia, severe hypertension, hyperthyroidism, pheochromocytoma or pregnancy, do not add vasoconstrictor to local anesthetic -Anatomic areas of risk -In patients with chronic use of corticosteroids. Protocol for minor surgery in anticoagulated patients - 3 Day Suspend Sintrom ® - 2 Day Suspend Sintrom ® and add subcutaneous LMWH - 1 Day Suspend Sintrom ® and add subcutaneous LMWH, single dose - 0 Day INR Control. If between 1 and 1.6 proceed to surgery. LMWH single subcutaneous dose. Patient will take the usual dose of Sintrom ® (the same as before the suspension). +1 Day LMWH single subcutaneous dose usual dose of Sintrom ® +2 Day usual dose of Sintrom ® +3 Day LMWH single subcutaneous dose. Usual dose of Sintrom ® +4 Day usual dose of Sintrom ® INR will be obtained on day +10 (seven days after surgery)

Table 3.
Precautions of minor surgery.

DOI: http://dx.doi.org/10.5772/intechopen.88811

uncooperative patients or refusal to sign the informed consent form is a contraindication for any minor surgery procedure or technique.

Direct oral anticoagulants [DOACs] (Dabigatran, Rivaroxaban, Apixaban, Edoxaban): If a moderate or high bleeding risk surgery, it can be omitted for approximately 2–3 days before a procedure, and resume 24 hours after surgery. However, cutaneous procedures (e.g., skin biopsy, tumor excision, bone marrow biopsy) generally considered to confer a low risk of bleeding [15].

6.2 Intraoperative complications

Vasovagal syncope is the most frequent complication and is more common in young men. Even some patients lose consciousness.

Treatment consists in administering oxygen and iv. fluids if needed and, in severe cases use atropine (0.5–1 mg sc or iv). Generally, most of patients recover spontaneously over a period of seconds to a few minutes.

6.3 Postoperative complications

- Infection can occur in up to 1% of minor surgical patients, symptoms such as fever and/or chills are only rarely seen. Infections are treated by removing some of the stitches, plus daily cleaning and disinfection of the wound and allowing the wound to close by secondary intention. If necessary an oral antibiotic regimen may be initiated and inserted drain into the wound.

- *Hematoma-seroma*: is paramount suturing the wound in layers with no gaps and, applying a compressive bandage to prevent their formation.

- *Wound dehiscence*: After wound dehiscence, repairs will take place by secondary intention.

- Hypertrophic scar and keloid scarring.

Conflict of interest

The authors declare no conflict of interest.

Author details

Jose Maria Arribas Blanco[1*], Wafa Elgeadi Saleh[2], Belén Chavero Méndez[2] and María Alvargonzalez Arrancudiaga[2]

1 Professor of Medicine Department, Faculty of Medicine, Universidad Autónoma de Madrid (UAM), Specialist in Family and Community Medicine, Madrid, Spain

2 Specialist in Family and Community Medicine, Servicio Madrileño de Salud (SERMAS), Madrid, Spain

*Address all correspondence to: jarribasb@gmail.com

References

[1] Arribas JM. Cirugía menor y procedimientos en medicina de familia. 2nd ed. Madrid: Jarpyo Editores; 2006

[2] Murphy R, Hague A, Srinivasan J. A review of forehead lipomas: Important tips for the training surgeon. The Surgeon. 2019;**17**:186

[3] Zuber TJ. Punch biopsy of the skin. American Family Physician. 2002;**65**(6):1155-1158, 1161-1162, 1164

[4] Freiman A, Bouganim N. History of cryotherapy. Dermatology Online Journal. 2005;**11**(2):9

[5] Hainer BL. Electrosurgery for the skin. American Family Physician. 2002;**66**(7):1259-1266

[6] Kudur MH, Pai SB, Sripathi H, Prabhu S. Sutures and suturing techniques in skin closure. Indian Journal of Dermatology, Venereology and Leprology. 2009;**75**(4):425-434

[7] Singer AJ, Quinn JV, Hollander JE. The cyanoacrylate topical skin adhesives. The American Journal of Emergency Medicine. 2008;**26**(4):490-496

[8] Hussain W, Mortimer NJ, Salmon PJ. Optimizing technique in elliptical excisional surgery: Some pearls for practice. The British Journal of Dermatology. 2009;**161**(3):697-698. Epub 2009 Jun 25

[9] Czarnowski C, Ponka D, Rughani R, Geoffrion P. Elliptical excision: Minor surgery video series. Canadian Family Physician. 2008;**54**(8):1144

[10] Wu T. Plastic surgery made easy—Simple techniques for closing skin defects and improving cosmetic results. Australian Family Physician. 2006;**35**(7):492-496

[11] Achar S, Kundu S. Principles of office anesthesia: Part I. Infiltrative anesthesia. American Family Physician. 2002;**66**(1):91-94

[12] Wolff K, Johnson RA. Fitzpatrick's Color Atlas and Synopsis of Clinical Dermatology. 6th ed. New York: El McGraw-Hill Companies, Inc; 2009

[13] Rahmani G, McCarthy P, Bergin D. The diagnostic accuracy of ultrasonography for soft tissue lipomas: A systematic review. Acta Radiologica Open. 2017;**6**:2058460117716704

[14] Wang YJ, Tang TY, Wang JY, et al. Genital basal cell carcinoma, a different pathogenesis from sun-exposed basal cell carcinoma? A case-control study of 30 cases. Journal of Cutaneous Pathology. 2018

[15] Beyer-Westendorf J, Gelbricht V, Förster K, et al. Peri-interventional management of novel oral anticoagulants in daily care: Results from the prospective Dresden NOAC registry. European Heart Journal. 2014;**35**:1888

Chapter 3

Approach to Chronic Urticaria from Primary Care and Emergency Services: Case Reports in Spain

Luis Geniz Rubio, Macarena Ávila Pérez, José Ángel López Díaz and Sara Alcántara Luna

Abstract

Urticaria is a common process. The true incidence is not known; it is believed that between 15 and 25% of the population may suffer at some point in his life. Acute urticaria has a prevalence of 20% and the chronic form 0.5–1%. Urticaria is a disease that affects the skin and mucosa, characterized by the presence of hives. It occurs as a localized intracutaneous edema circled and an area of redness (erythema), which is typically itchy. There are histaminergic foods and drugs that worsen the prognosis of the disease. Foods which rely on aging to taste nice are always presumed to be high in histamine (chocolate, yogurt, seafood, strawberries, etc.) and drugs like nonsteroidal anti-inflammatory drugs. For diagnosis we have several tools (urticarial activity score, chronic urticaria quality-of-life questionnaire (CU-Q2oL), urticaria control test, etc., among which the most useful, simple, and cost-effective is the clinic history). The treatment of choice are antihistamines, from a daily tablet up to four tablets as maximum dose. Corticosteroids are excluded to exacerbations and must be prescribed in short guideline (maximum 10 days) without progressive decrease. Severe forms of urticaria resistant to treatment with antihistamines are treated with biological agents like omalizumab.

Keywords: urticaria, hives, itching, angioedema, antihistamines

1. Introduction

The interest in making this chapter was to explain the pathology of chronic urticaria as prevalent and its high morbidity.

We often see this problem in our primary care consultations and emergency services, so we consider its important to make a chapter about urticaria.

The current version of the EAACI/GA^{2}LEN/EDF/WAO urticaria guideline from 2018 contains new aspects about diagnosis and treatment.

At the end of the chapter, we show a series of cases treated in our practice (observed in a Juan Ramon Jimenez's dermatology room in Huelva, Spain), exposing results obtained with the different forms of treatment (**Figure 1**).

IntechOpen

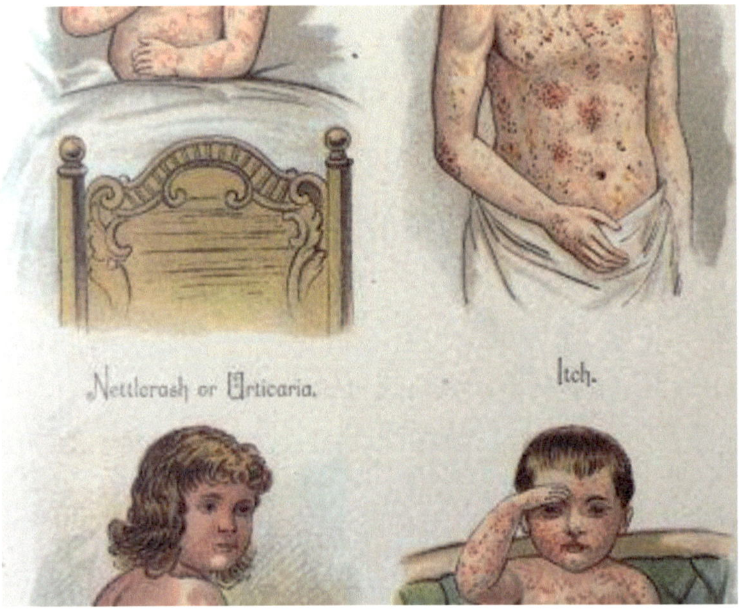

Figure 1.
Chronic urticaria.

2. Epidemiology

Urticaria is a common process. Although the true incidence is not known, it is believed that between 15 and 25% of the population may suffer at some point in his life. Acute urticaria has a prevalence of 20% and the chronic form 0.5–1% [1]. Age, race, sex, occupation, geographical region, and the season of the year may be implicated in urticaria and angioedema. The majority of acute episodes are due to adverse reactions to medications or food or, in children, to viral diseases.

Spontaneous chronic urticaria represents about 70% of all chronic hives and may persist for several years. Patients with chronic urticaria often describe a decrease in the quality of life because of itching and may have alterations of sleep, fatigue, social isolation, or emotional disorders (**Figures 2–4**).

2.1 Physiopathology

Urticaria is a disease that affects the skin and mucosa, characterized by the presence of hives. It is a localized intracutaneous edema that circled an area of redness (erythema), which is typically itchy. Individual hives can persist from 30 minutes to 36 hours and can measure from only 1 millimeter up to 15–20 cm in diameter, named giant hives [2]. Increased dilation and permeability of blood vessels that characterize the hives are present in the superficial dermis and undertake the venous plexus located there (**Figure 5**). It is rare and it may occur with concomitant angioedema.

Another similar entity is angioedema, with a similar mechanism as urticaria [3], but the pathology is located in the deep dermis and subcutaneous tissue, and swelling is the main manifestation. The skin may be normal or erythematous. There is less itching, but it can cause pain or burning sensation. The mouth, lips, eyes, throat, feet, and hands are most commonly affected (**Figures 6** and 7). When angioedema affects the throat, it can be life-threatening, because there is interference in

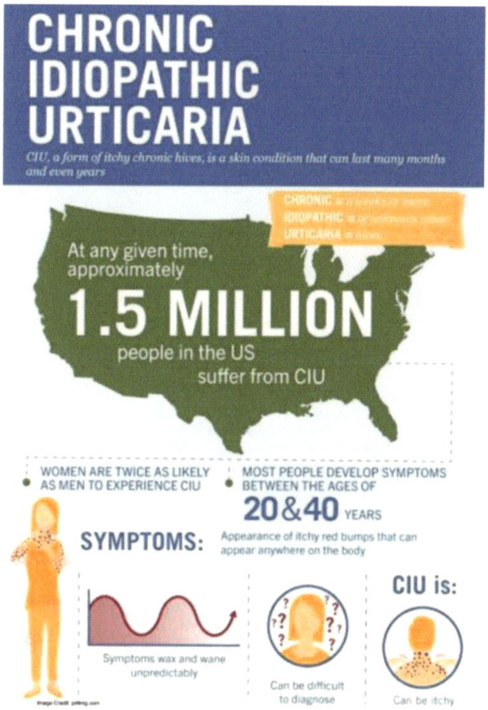

Figure 2.
Epidemiology of chronic urticaria in United States.

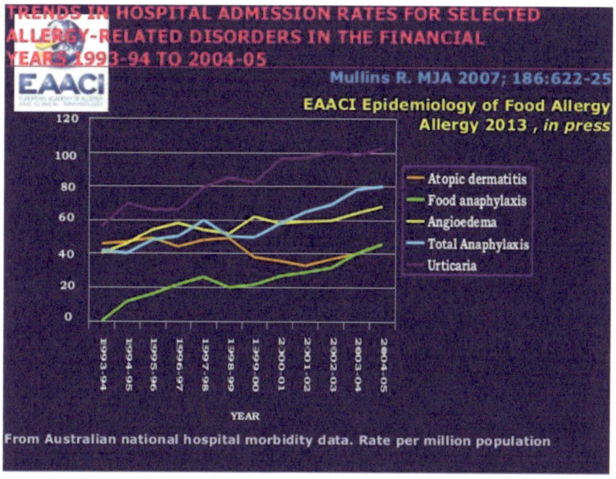

Figure 3.
Epidemiology of chronic urticaria in Australia.

breathing. It is caused by an allergic reaction, sometimes by a hereditary condition (hereditary angioedema), but normally we do not know the cause [3].

2.2 Food histamine liberator

Foods that require a ripening process to achieve a better taste are presumed to have a high histamine content. In the same way as foods that are made during fermentation. These include de following [4] (**Table 1**).

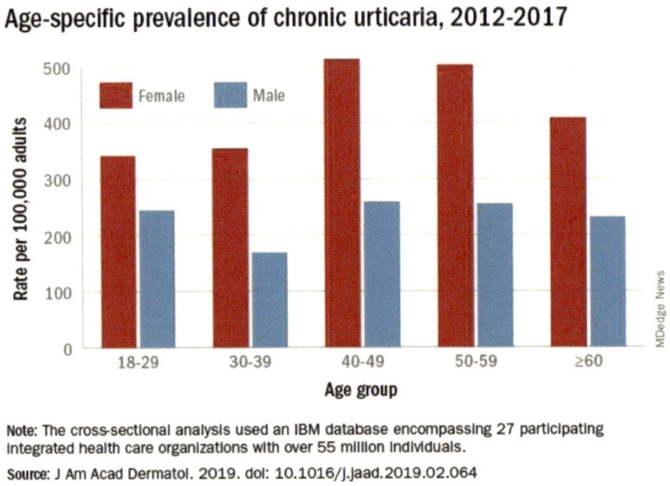

Figure 4.
Prevalence of chronic urticaria.

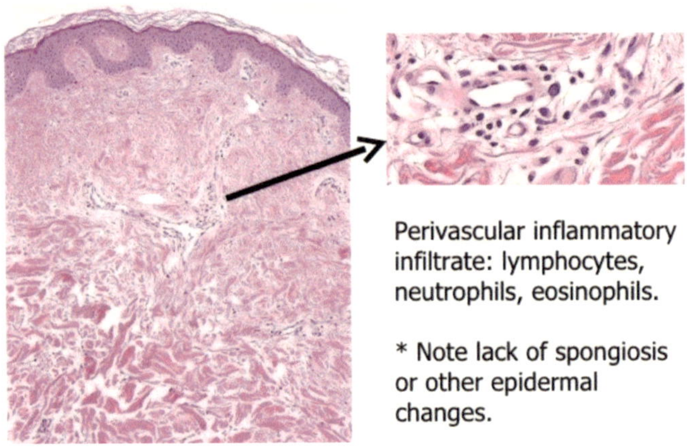

Figure 5.
Urticaria. Picture with histological findings.

The Spanish society of diamine oxidase (DAO) states on their website that the following food histamine liberators:

- Alcohol, citrus fruits, strawberries, pineapple, kiwi, tomato sauce, seafood, chocolate, fish, mushrooms, pig, cereals, and egg white.

- Some food additives such as glutamate, benzoate, several colorants (yellow E-102 and E-110, E-124, amaranth E-123), sulfites, and nitrites can release endogenous histamine.

The department for dermatology in Bonn's paper lists the following foods as being capable of releasing endogenous histamine (**Table 2**).

2.3 Pathogenesis

The mast cell is the main effector cell in urticaria and angioedema. Cutaneous mast cells attach to fibronectin and laminin through the integrin beta1 of Very Late

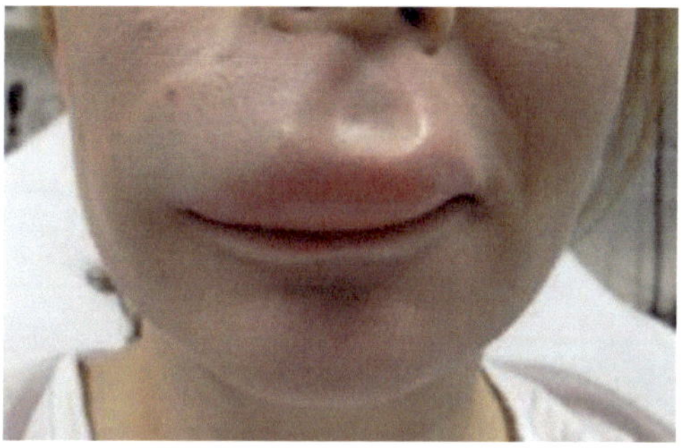

Figure 6.
Angioedema.

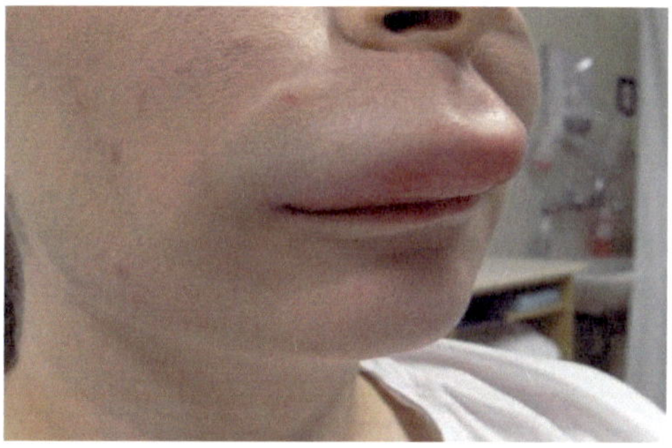

Figure 7.
Angioedema.

Yogurt	Soured cream
Buttermilk	Quark
Cottage cheese	Alcohol
Hard cheeses, cheddar	Vinegar
Aged cheeses, brie	Sauerkraut

Table 1.
Histamine liberator food.

Antigen (VLA), VLA-3, VLA-4, and VLA-5 activation and vitronectin through alfa1 and beta3 integrin [5].

Once activated, the mast cell releases granules containing histamine and other mediators of inflammation such as platelet activating factor (PAF) from, TNF alpha, IL-3, IL-4, IL-5, IL-6, IL-8, IL-13, GM-CSF, PGD-2, and leukotrienes (LTC4, LTD4, LTEA). Histamine, TNF alpha, and IL-8 also stimulate endothelial adhesion molecules that favors the migration of eosinophils, monocytes, and neutrophils from the bloodstream to the skin.

Histamine is an amine vasoactive located in granules of mast cells [5], basophils, and platelets. Its effects on the skin are mediated through histamine H1 and H2 receptors. H1 receptors mediate urticaria vasodilation, increased vascular permeability, and sensory nerve stimulation. Sensory nerve stimulation determines the release of neuropeptides such as substance P, peptide vasoactive intestinal (VIP), and somatostatin, which in turn induce the mast cell activation and increase in histamine.

Citrus fruit	Chocolate
Papaya	Fish
Strawberries	Crustaceans
Pineapple	Pork
Nuts	Egg white
Peanuts	Additives
Tomatoes	Liquorice
Spinach	Spices

Table 2.
Foods as being capable of releasing endogenous histamine.

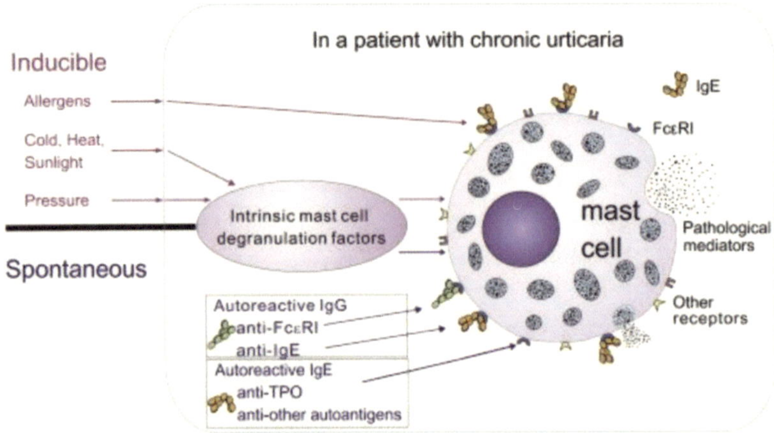

Figure 8.
Physiopathology of urticaria. Note like that the mast cells are the principal cells implicated.

The vascular endothelium expressed a significant number of H2 receptors, so the vascular response in the UC is an immunomodulatory effect, to increase the synthesis of pro-inflammatory cytokines such as IL-1 and IL-6 of monocytes and IL-6 and IL-8 cell endothelial. In addition to histamine, other soluble factors synthesized by mast cells contribute to the increase of vascular dilation and permeability; favor chemotaxis, cell activation of leukocyte, and endothelial cells; and induce stimulation sensory. These are the cytokines, chemokines, and neuropeptides and arachidonic acid metabolites.

The degranulation is attributed to immunological causes (autoimmune, IgE-dependent, immune complexes, complement-dependent), not immune (pseudoallergies, agents release by mast cells) and idiopathic. The path of the synthesis of prostaglandins and leukotrienes, hours later the mast cell activation, occurs in the synthesis of leukotrienes and prostaglandins from arachidonic acid via two-way enzymatic metabolism: the cyclooxygenase path and the lipoxygenase pathways.

Studies have shown that LTB4 has a potent chemotactic activity, which is produced by mast cells in the early and selective recruitment of leukocytes. At chronic urticaria (CU), these mediators appear to be the most important in the chronicity of the disease. There are no immune reactions (pseudoallergics); the mechanisms are not clear but may compromise the metabolism of arachidonic acid, prostaglandins, and leukotrienes [2] (**Figure 8**).

DOI: http://dx.doi.org/10.5772/intechopen.88369

3. Classification

According to the time evolution, urticaria can be divided into:

- Acute urticaria: less than 6 weeks.

- Chronic urticaria*: lesions appear for more than 6 weeks [6].

Recurrent urticaria: outbreaks recur over time, but its duration is limited. Episodes of hives last less than asymptomatic intervals.

* Chronic urticaria is divided into two:

Spontaneous chronic urticaria: spontaneous emergence of hives, angioedema, or both for longer than 6 weeks, due to a known or unknown cause.

Inducible urticaria: physical urticarial (This hives occur at the site of the stimulation)l, cholinergic, aquagenic and contact urticarias (**Figure 9**).

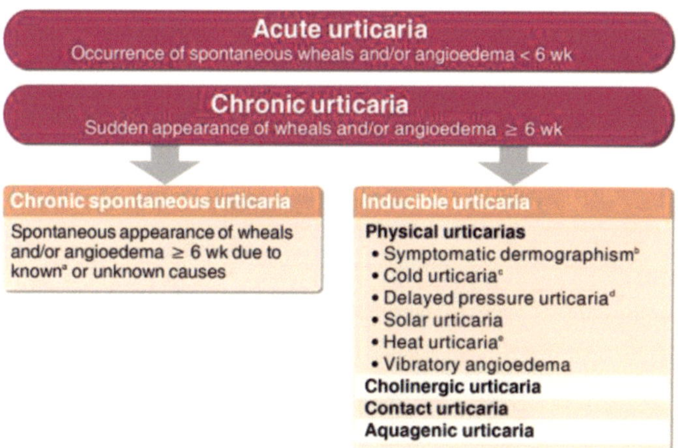

Figure 9.
Acute and chronic urticaria.

4. Symptomatology

Urticaria typically presents well circumscribed wheals (polimorphyc, serpenginous or round), with intensely pruritic for less than 24 hours of evolution. Wheals can be generalized, including arms, legs, face. Urticaria +/− angioedema (primarily in the face), can be acute (with an evolution of less than 6 weeks), or chronic (greater than 6 weeks [7] (**Figures 10–15**).

5. Diagnosis

For diagnosis we have several tools, among which the most useful, simple, and cost-effective is the clinical history, but we can ask for additional tests in the case of diagnostic doubt or suspicion of systemic disease [8].

5.1 Clinical history

A detailed clinical history and a good physical examination of the patient are necessary to make the diagnosis.

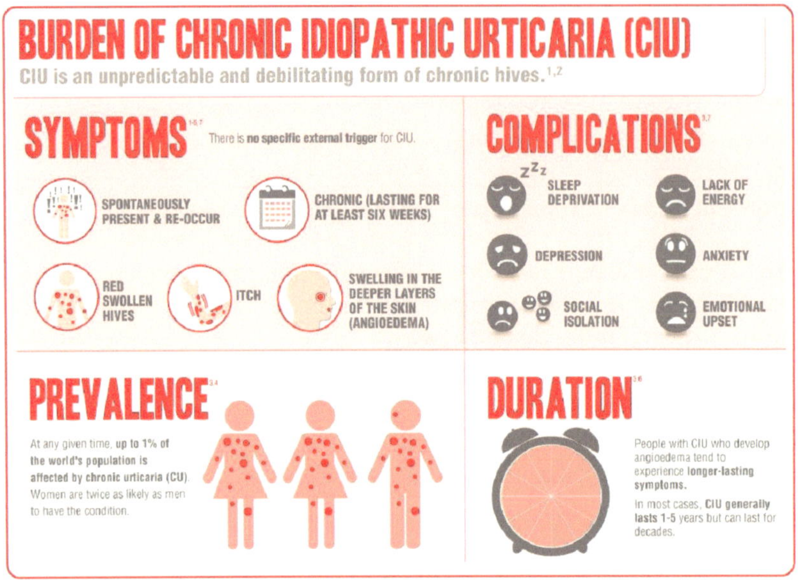

Figure 10.
Generalities of urticaria.

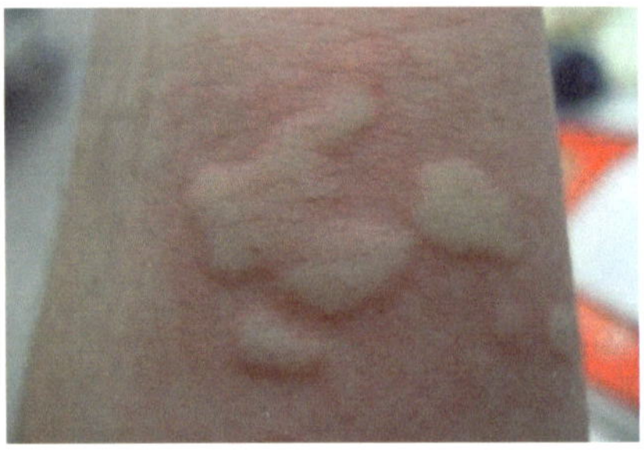

Figure 11.
Dermatological manifestations of urticaria. Note the typical hives.

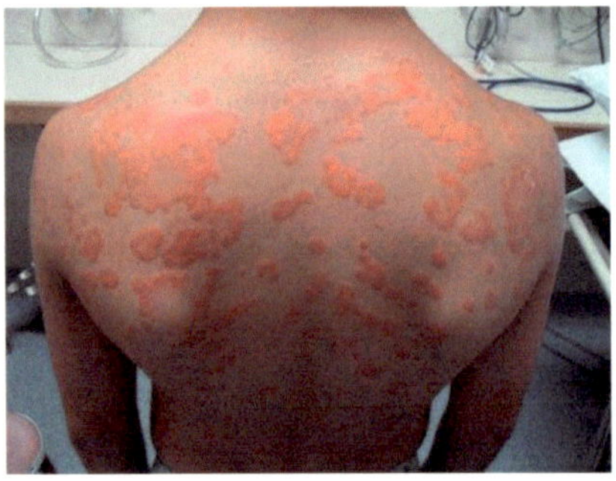

Figure 12.
Dermatological manifestations of urticaria. Note the erythema.

Thanks to its history, we can classify chronic urticaria as spontaneous or inducible. For this, we must focus on the following aspects:

- A family history of atopy or urticaria.
- Commonly used drugs and relation with the hives.

- A history of allergies, infections, or any other cause that has been able to trigger hives.
- Work performed and hobbies.
- Induction of urticaria due to exercise or exposure to physical agents.
- How the body reacts to insect bites.
- If the patient has been on holidays or trip recently.
- If it has relationship with the menstrual cycle or stress.
- If the quality of life is affected.
- Duration of the disease.
- Frequency and duration of the hives, size, shape, and distribution.
- If associated symptoms are subjective such as pain, burning, etc.
- If the patient has nocturnal or diurnal variation.
- How the response was to the treatments used.

5.2 Complementary tests

Complementary tests serve as support to the diagnosis, to detect associated systemic diseases or for differential diagnosis.

Basic laboratory tests, as blood count and biochemical reaction (determination of C-reactive protein, glomerular sedimentation rate), can help us rule out there is a systemic disease. The baseline of tryptase, antithyroid antibodies, and thyroid profile and study of complement and specific IgE where allergy is suspected, could also be useful. If an infection cause is suspected, hepatitis B and C virus or Helicobacter Pylori could be detected.

New guidelines recommend not to perform additional exploration in a systematic way in acute urticaria and just a complete blood count with ESR and a suspension of nonsteroidal anti inflammatory drugs (NSAIDs) in the CU (**Figure 16**).

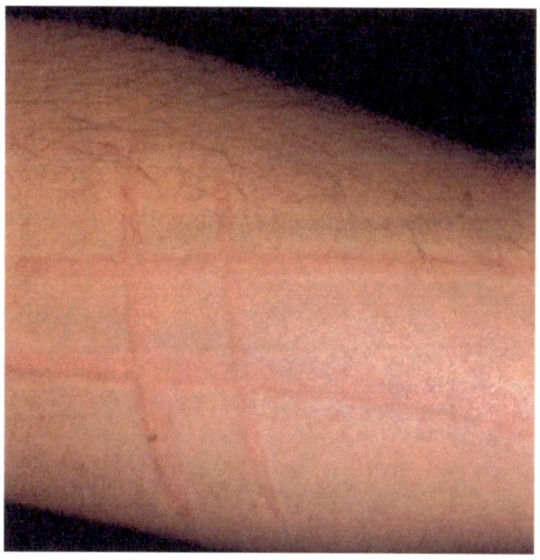

Figure 13.
Linear hives made by compression.

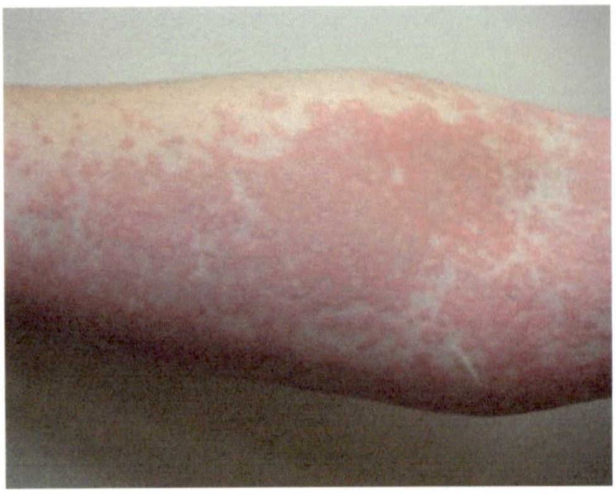

Figure 14.
Coalescing urticarial papules.

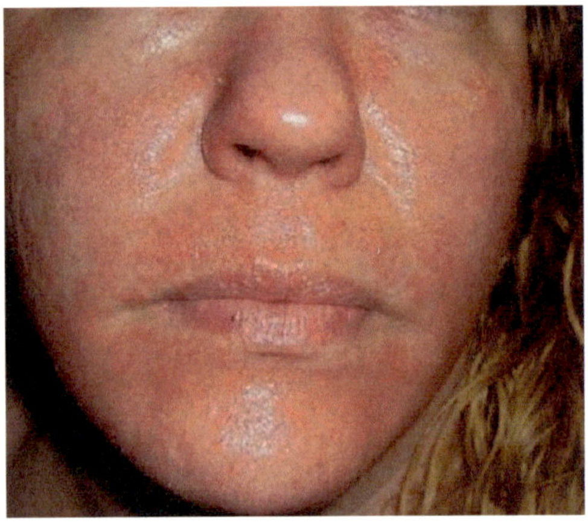

Figure 15.
Urticaria and angioedema.

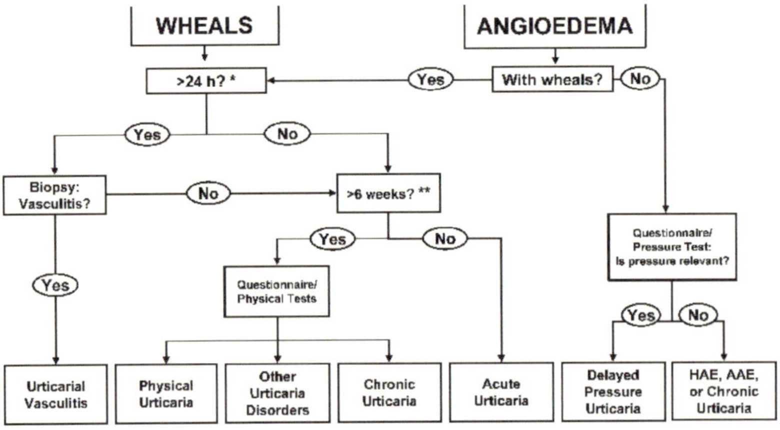

Figure 16.
Diagnosis algorithm.

6. Treatment

Different ways are approached for the treatment of urticaria: eliminating histaminergic food such as seafoods, canned goods, tomatoes, strawberries, bananas, pineapple, or apples and avoiding nonsteroidal anti-inflammatory drugs (NSAIDs) [9], nonsedative H1-antihistamines, and in severe cases systemic corticosteroids [10].

6.1 Mild forms of urticaria

- The treatment of choice are antihistamines, from a daily tablet up to four tablets as maximum dose.
- Corticosteroids are excluded for exacerbations and must be prescribed in short guideline (maximum 10 days) without progressive decrease.
- Avoid taking NSAIDs.

6.2 Severe forms of urticaria or exacerbations and associated angioedema

- Nonsedative H1-antihistamines to full dose (four tablets in a day) [11].
- Systemic corticoids, preferably in short treatment (10-day short guideline).
- Forms resistant to treatment: biological agents (omalizumab*).
- Avoid taking NSAIDs (**Figure 17**).

*Omalizumab is a recombinant humanized monoclonal antibody, which blocks the high-affinity Fc receptor of IgE (**Figure 18**). It has been approved for treatment in cases of moderate-to-severe asthma, but it has promising results in the management also of chronic urticaria [12]. The dose is 150 or 300 mg by subcutaneous injection every 4 weeks. Dosing is not dependent on body weight or serum IgE level. The appropriate duration for CIU has not been evaluated yet. It's necessary to periodically reassess the need for continued therapy with omalizumab [13].

6.2.1 Clinical guidelines

The European Academy of Allergy and Clinical Immunology (EAACI)/Global Allergy and Asthma European Network (GA2LEN)/European Dermatology Forum (EDF)/World Allergy Organization (WAO) and the American Academy of Allergy, Asthma, and Immunology (AAAAI) have some differences in their recommendations for urticaria treatment, but the core recommendations remain similar.

A brief summary of *AAAAI guidelines* are as follows [14]:

As first-line treatment, second-generation nonsedating H1 antihistamines.

Remain in the treatment algorithm first-generation H 1 antihistamines (differs from EAACI/GA 2LEN/EDF/WAO guidelines).

Second-line options to consider: adding other second-generation H 1 antihistamines, up-dosing second-generation H 1 antihistamines, leukotriene receptor

Efficacy of increased doses of non-sedating antihistamines in patients with chronic urticaria

Author ref	Drug	Dose (mg)	Efficacy Responders/n	%
Finn [17]	Fexofenadine	120 BD	46/89	51.6
Finn [17]	Fexofenadine	240 BD	54/83	64.9
Nelson [18]	Fexofenadine	120 BD	33/77	42.8
Nelson [18]	Fexofenadine	240 BD	46/82	56.0
Giménez-Arnau [19]	Rupatadine	20 QD	69/109	63.3
Dubertret [20]	Rupatadine	20 QD	48/67	71.6
Siebenhaar [21]	Desloratadine	20 QD	15/30	50.0
Staevska [22]	Desloratadine	10 QD	7/36	19.4
Staevska [22]	Desloratadine	20 QD	1/29	3.4
Staevska [22]	Levocetirizine	10 QD	8/31	25.8
Staevska [22]	Levocetirizine	20 QD	5/23	21.7
Krause [23]	Bilastine	40 QD	11/20	55.0
Krause [23]	Bilastine	80 QD	12/20	60.0

Figure 17.
Nonsedative antihistamines.

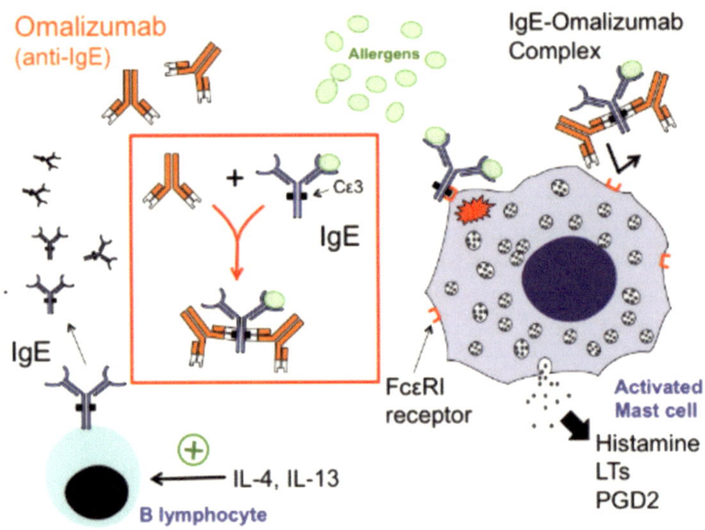

Figure 18.
*Monoclonal antibody that binds to the Cε3 domain of circulating IgE, which prevents IgE from binding to and activating receptors in mast cells (***Figure 19***).*

antagonists, adding H 2 antagonists or first-generation H 1 antihistamines at bedtime.

Omalizumab as third-line treatment.

Corticosteroids considered only for short treatment.

Cyclosporine A* is used in refractory chronic urticaria not responsive to other treatments.

A brief summary of *EAACI/GA2LEN/EDF/WAO guidelines* are as follows:

First-line treatment, second-generation H 1 antihistamines.

Up-dosing second-generation H1 antihistamines are the second-line therapy.

Omalizumab is the third-line treatment, which is recommended because it is less toxic than cyclosporine A.

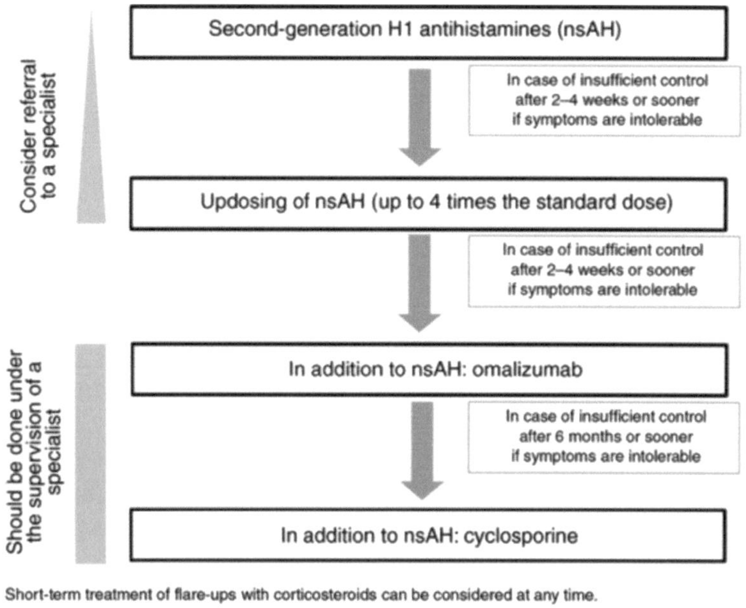

Figure 19.
Recommended treatment algorithm for chronic urticaria.

Not included in algorithm H2 antihistamines (used only on an individual case).

Avoid first-generation H1 antihistamines based on benefit to risk ratio.

Corticosteroids may be considered only for the short-term intervention.

Cyclosporine A for refractory chronic urticaria not responsive to other treatments.

*Cyclosporin A is an immunosuppressive agent, widely used in organ transplantation to prevent rejection.

The current version of the *EAACI/GA^{2}LEN/EDF/WAO urticaria guideline* recommends:

When chronic inducible urticaria is suspected, differential diagnoses should be ruled out. The diagnosis should be confirmed by provocation test disease. The activity should be measured by determining the trigger threshold disease burden and control should be measured.

Second-generation H1 antihistamines remain the treatment of first choice.

If continuous treatment for 2–4 weeks does not lead to adequate control of symptoms, the guidelines recommend up-dosing (up to four times the standard dose).

If there is no improvement with high-dose antihistamines, it is recommended to add omalizumab to the regimen in patients with chronic spontaneous urticaria.

If there is no success after 6 months of omalizumab therapy, off-label treatment with cyclosporine is recommended.

7. Assessment scales

Assessment scales serve to evaluate the treatment, as well as this pathological entity affects the quality of life of the patient. We have the urticarial activity score (UAS) [15] or angioedema activity score (AAS) [16], chronic urticaria quality-of-life questionnaire, and urticaria control test (UCT).

Score	Wheals	Pruritus
0	None	None
1	Mild (<20 wheals/24 h)	Mild (present but not annoying or troublesome)
2	Moderate(20-50 wheals/24 h)	Moderate (troublesome but does not interfere with normal daily activity or sleep
3	Intense (>50 wheals/24 h or large confluent areas of wheals)	Intense (severe pruritus, which is sufficiently troublesome to interfere with normal daily activity or sleep)

Sum of score: 0–6.

Figure 20.
UAS.

Urticaria control test

Name: ____________________ Date: ___ . ___ . ______

Date of birth: _____ . ____ . ______

Instructions: You have hives (urticaria). The following questions are meant to assess the current disease status. Please read each question carefully and select the one answer that *best describes your situation.* Please refer to the *past 4 weeks. Don't ponder for too long and remember to answer all questions* and to select *only one answer* for each question.

1. To what extent have you suffered from **physical symptoms of urticaria (pruritus, wheals and/or swelling)** in the past 4 weeks?
   O very severely O severely O moderately O slightly O not at all
2. How much has your **quality of life** been affected by the urticaria in the past 4 weeks?
   O very severely O severely O moderately O slightly O not at all
3. How often has the **treatment** of your urticaria **not been sufficient** to control the urticaria symptoms in the past 4 weeks?
   O very frequently O frequently O occasionally O rarely O not at all
4. How well has your urticaria been **under control overall** in the past 4 weeks?
   O not at all O hardly O moderately O well O completely

Figure 21.
Urticaria control test.

The current guideline endorses the urticaria activity score and/or the angioedema activity score to assess the disease activity in CSU patients [17] (**Figure 20**).

The urticaria control test should be used in all CSU patients. The UCT is a retrospective tool used to rapidly and reliably assess disease control with four simple questions (**Figure 21**). Patients answer each of the four UCT questions, and the corresponding points (0–4 per answer) are added up to yield a total score of 0–16. The cutoff for controlled urticaria is 12 points. A score of 11 or less indicates insufficient disease control, whereas a score of 12 or more suggests adequate disease control [18].

Conflict of interest

None.

Thanks

We want to thank IntechOpen for the opportunity to publish this chapter. We also want to thank our friends and family for their patience and unconditional support.

Author details

Luis Geniz Rubio[1*], Macarena Ávila Pérez[2], José Ángel López Díaz[1] and Sara Alcántara Luna[1]

1 Hospital Juan Ramón Jimenez, Huelva, Spain

2 Hospital Reina Sofía, Córdoba, Spain

*Address all correspondence to: luis.geniz@gmail.com

References

[1] Zuberbier T et al. The EAACI/GA(2) LEN/EDF/WAO guideline for the definition, classification, diagnosis, and management of urticaria: The 2013 revision and update. Allergy. 2014;**69**(7):868-887

[2] Greaves MW. Pathology and classification of urticaria. Immunology and Allergy Clinics of North America. 2014;**34**(1):1-9

[3] Maurer M, Magerl M, Metz M, et al. Practical algorithm for diagnosing patients with recurrent wheals or angioedema. Allergy. 2013;**68**:816-819

[4] Zuberbier T. The role of allergens and pseudoallergens in urticaria. The Journal of Investigative Dermatology. Symposium Proceedings. 2001;**6**:132-134

[5] Church MK, Kolkhir P, Metz M, Maurer M. The role and relevance of mast cells in urticaria. Immunological Reviews. 2018;**282**:232-247

[6] Bernstein JA, Lang MD, Khan DA. The diagnosis and management of acute and chronic urticaria: 2014 update. The Journal of Allergy and Clinical Immunology. 2014;**133**:1270-1277

[7] Kulthanan K. Clinical practice guideline for diagnosis and management of urticaria. Asian Pacific Journal of Allergy and Immunology. 2016;**34**(3):190-200

[8] Zuberbier T, Aberer W, Asero R, et al. The EAACI/GA 2LEN/EDF/WAO guideline for the definition, classification, diagnosis and management of urticaria. The 2017 revision and update. Allergy. 2018;**73**:1393-1414

[9] Guillén-Aguinaga S, Jáuregui Presa I, Aguinaga-Ontoso E, et al. Updosing nonsedating antihistamines in patients with chronic spontaneous urticaria: A systematic review and meta-analysis. The British Journal of Dermatology. 2016;**175**:1153-1165

[10] Sánchez-Borges M, Ansotegui I, Montero Jimenez J, et al. Comparative efficacy of non-sedating antihistamine updosing in patients with chronic urticaria. World Allergy Organization Journal. 2014;**7**(1):33

[11] Maurer M, Staubach P, Raap U, et al. H1-antihistamine-refractory chronic spontaneous urticaria: It's worse than we thought–first results of the multicenter real-life AWARE study. Clinical and Experimental Allergy. 2017;**47**:684-692

[12] Maurer M, Metz M, Brehler R, et al. Omalizumab treatment in patients with chronic inducible urticaria: A systematic review of published evidence. The Journal of Allergy and Clinical Immunology. 2018;**141**:638-649

[13] Kaplan A, Ledford D, Ashby M, et al. Omalizumab in patients with symptomatic chronic idiopathic/spontaneous urticaria despite standard combination therapy. The Journal of Allergy and Clinical Immunology. 2013;**132**:101-109

[14] Diakow M, James W. Chronic Urticaria Guidelines. Available in emedicine. Medscape. Article 1050052; 2017

[15] Hawro T, Ohanyan T, Schoepke N, et al. The urticaria activity score—Validity, reliability, and responsiveness. The Journal of Allergy and Clinical Immunology. In Practice. 2018;**6**:1185-1190

[16] Weller K, Magerl M, Peveling-Oberhag A, et al. The angioedema quality of life questionnaire

(AE-QoL)-assessment of sensitivity to change and minimal clinically important difference. Allergy. 2016;**71**:1203-1209

[17] Mathias SD, Crosby RD, Zazzali JL, et al. Evaluating the minimally important difference of the urticaria activity score and other measures of disease activity in patients with chronic idiopathic urticari. Annals of Allergy, Asthma and Immunology. 2012;**108**:20-24

[18] Weller K, Groffik A, Church MK, et al. Development and validation of the urticaria control test: A patient-reported outcome instrument for assessing urticaria control. The Journal of Allergy and Clinical Immunology. 2014;**133**:1365-1372

Chapter 4

Cultural Adaptation of a Cardiovascular Health Education Program among Hypertensive Primary Care Patients from Rural Nigeria

Aina Olufemi Odusola and Ayoade Adedokun

Abstract

Culturally adapted behavioral treatments can optimize care. Following standard guidelines we adapted and tested a hypertension education program among primary care patients with hypertension from rural Nigeria. We reviewed literature and collected qualitative information from hypertensive patients to implement the first three of five cultural adaptation stages: *Information gathering, Adaptation design, and Preliminary adaptation testing*. Information obtained was used to adapt a *Cardiovascular Health Education Program* (CHEP) from a similar program *Culturally Appropriate Hypertension Education* (CAHE). CHEP was evaluated among 149 hypertensive patients using pre, – post design, and performance of behavioral goals. Data were analyzed using descriptive statistics and thematic contents. CHEP retained essential features of CAHE and added new culturally relevant information. Local context factors like substitutability of dietary *salt* and exercisability with cultural activities motivated healthy behavior and enhanced cultural fitness. Culturally permissive unhealthy practices were discouraged; intentional weight gain (*big is beautiful*), and non-smoking tobacco use (*sniffing, licking*). Performance of behavioral goals was outstanding; over 60% practiced self-set goals effectively. Standard cultural adaptation of behavioral education program demonstrated potential to limit cardiovascular diseases among hypertensive patients. Guideline-based culturally adapted intervention increased hypertension self-management capabilities among hypertensive primary care patients from rural Nigeria.

Keywords: standardized cultural adaptation, behavioral health education, goal setting assessment, hypertension self-management, rural Nigeria

1. Introduction

Hypertension is a major risk factor of cardiovascular diseases (CVD), and is highly prevalent in sub-Saharan Africa (SSA) [1, 2]. CVD including ischemic heart disease and stroke are the world's biggest killers, having killed 15.2 million people in 2016 alone [3], and being responsible for 17.9 million (31%) of global deaths annually [4]. To limit CVD, World health organization (WHO) advocated preventive management of hypertension and other CVD risk factors [4]. In Nigeria where the age-standardized prevalence of Hypertension is 19.3%, only 8% of hypertensive patients are aware, 3% controlled and just 5% are covered by treatment [5]. Fortunately though, willingness to adopt recommended lifestyle measures is encouraging among hypertensive patients [6].

In African rural settings deep-routed cultural orientations can manifest in beliefs and perceptions about health that vary with modern medical perceptions. It is beneficial to re-orientate people in such deeply cultural settings to acquire well informed modern health perspectives. This can be achieved by introducing culturally appropriate behavioral health interventions that have undergone cultural adaptation based on the people's traditional health practices and cultural beliefs.

Cultural adaptation is the systematic process of increasing cultural content and cultural sensitivity of existing behavioral treatments to effectively address distinct sub-cultural group needs. *Cultural sensitivity* has been defined in two dimensions: 1) surface structure elements; and 2) deep structure elements. While *Surface Structure elements* refer to the matching of intervention materials to observable superficial cultural characteristics of a target population e.g. music, food, places, dressing, language etc., *Deep Structure elements* refer to the use of cultural, historical, environmental and social norms and practices to modify targeted health behavior among a target population [7, 8].

An ideal behavioral treatment intervention should be adapted culturally by following standard procedures. Studies have shown that guideline-based cultural adaptation process has potential to increase acceptability, attractiveness and effectiveness of treatment support programs among target populations [9–11]. Furthermore evidence abounds that systematic cultural adaptation of behavioral treatments offer intrinsic self-efficacy benefits for patients [12–14]. Reports further suggests that cultural adaptation of health interventions can enhance service delivery when implemented as a living process with dynamism for continuous feedback, replicability and improvement [11]. Conversely other interventions that are not culturally adapted can unwittingly discourage uptake of recommended lifestyles by patients at risk of CVD [15]. Systematic review evidence from global perspective have also highlighted usefulness of culturally adapted interventions in control of CVD risk factors [16]. Currently however, there is a dearth of regional studies investigating usefulness and exploitability of cultural adaptation of treatment interventions in SSA settings.

To implement standard cultural adaptation, Barrera et al. identified five guideline-based sequential stages involved from a Consensus on Updates of Models for Effective Cultural Adaptation as follows: *Information Gathering (stage one)*, *Preliminary Adaptation Design (stage two)*, *Preliminary Adaptation Testing (stage three)*, *Adaptation Refinement (stage four)*, and *Cultural Adaptation Trial (stage five)* [10]. There is however a need for continuous improvement in the adaptation development process as issues and challenges were recently reported on emerging multistep frameworks design of cultural adaptation process, suggesting need for further research to conclude on effectiveness of interventions adapted based on such designs [17].

The effectiveness of culturally adapted interventions can be evaluated using standard testing procedures. Studies suggest that goal setting and pursuance among patients can be effective in promoting acculturation and adoption of adapted interventions among populations at risk of CVD. Similar evidence abounds that goal setting is useful in evaluating effectiveness of culturally adapted interventions including acquisition of behavioral self-management skills [18–21]. Indeed the setting and pursuing of culturally adapted goals to stimulate healthy behavior have enhanced chronic disease self-management skills [18, 20]. Available evidence further suggests that the more frequently goals are set and pursued, the easier and faster patients learn and acquire targeted self-management skills [19].

In this study, following standard guidelines and procedures we culturally adapted an existing hypertension education program to produce a similar variant with enhanced cultural content and sensitivity using the first three out of five sequential steps. We proceeded further to evaluate the adapted program for *cultural-fitness* using patients' performance of set behavioral goals, and for *effectiveness* using hypertension treatment outcomes.

2. Methods

2.1 Background to study design

A mixed methods study in two phases: in *phase 1* we conducted qualitative study to adapt a *Cardiovascular Health Education Program* (CHEP) from a similar *Culturally Appropriate Hypertension Education* (CAHE) program; while in *phase 2* we used quantitative and observational designs to evaluate the adapted CHEP for effectiveness and cultural fitness. **Figure 1** shows relationships between various phases of the adaptation process. The cultural adaptation process involved *formative* and *construction arms*. In the *formative arm* we collected information from literature and from qualitative interviews with 40 hypertensive patients to develop the original form and content of CHEP [22, 23]. In the *construction arm* we used information from the *formative arm* to supplement protocol and materials originally developed for CAHE by Beune et al. [24], to increase cultural sensitivity of CHEP for specific needs of hypertensive patients from Nigeria. CAHE was previously developed in the Netherlands to support treatment adherence and BP control among Afro-Surinamese and Ghanaian primary care patients with hypertension [24, 25]. Similarly, CHEP was the main outcome of a cardiovascular disease (CVD) prevention project, *Quality Improvement Cardiovascular Care Kwara* (QUICK-2) in rural Nigeria [26]. The goal of QUICK-2 was to develop and evaluate a patient-centered cardiovascular health education program to increase adherence to prescribed pharmacologic treatment and healthy behavior among hypertensive patients. QUICK-2 was implemented in two consecutive parts: *development of CHEP* over

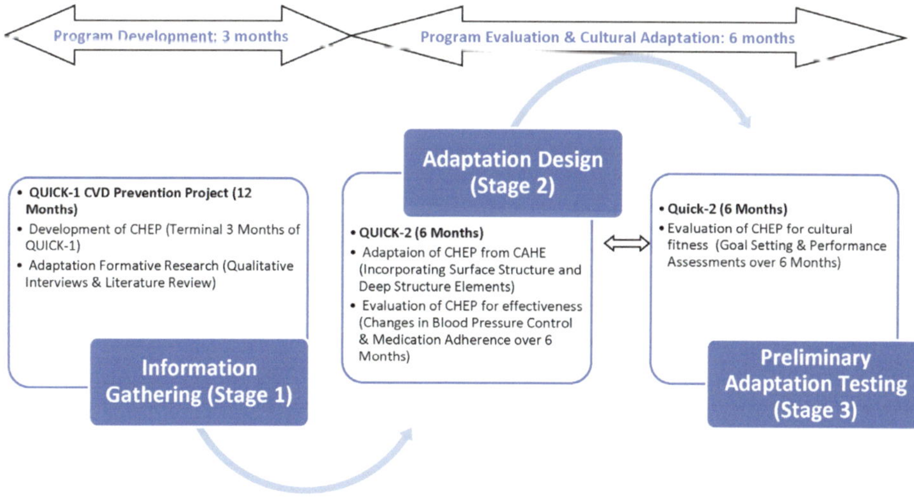

Figure 1.
Cultural adaptation study in relation to QUICK-1 and QUICK-2 studies.

3 months (*part 1*), and *evaluation of CHEP* over the subsequent 6 months (*part 2*). Prior to this, QUICK-2 was preceded by a related QUICK-1 study over 12 months, to assess feasibility of providing quality CVD prevention care to 349 hypertensive patients enrolled in a community-based health insurance program in Kwara state, Nigeria [27]. At the end of QUICK-1, 149 of the 349 participants did not meet hypertension control targets despite accessing standard, quality CVD prevention care of QUICK-1. The 149 uncontrolled patients consequently met criteria for inclusion in QUICK-2. We had hypothesized that 'consulting room' health education made available to the patients during 'usual hypertension care' in QUICK-1 was inadequate to support adherence and improve treatment outcome. We therefore developed CHEP to improve adherence and outcome among the uncontrolled patients during QUICK-2 [13].

In the current study, our focus is to describe the *processes and stages* involved in cultural adaptation of CHEP from CAHE and the testing of adapted CHEP for cultural fitness, namely *Information Gathering (stage 1), Preliminary Adaptation Design (stage 2), and Preliminary Adaptation Testing (stage 3)*. A CHEP effectiveness control trial would be implemented in future using two final stages: *Adaptation Refinement (stage 4)*, and *Cultural Adaptation Trial (stage 5)*.

2.1.1 Study setting

Our study was implemented at a primary healthcare center, *Ogo Oluwa Hospital* (OOH) in the sleepy agrarian rural town, Bacita in Edu local government area of Kwara state, north central Nigeria. At that time OOH was a provider in the Dutch government funded Kwara State Health Insurance (KSHI) program [28], http://hifund.org/. Bacita was inhabited by mainly Nupe and Yoruba ethnic groups in addition to pockets of few other Nigerian tribes. The predominant occupations in the region were artisanship, farming, petty trading and fishing.

In the following section we describe the steps taken in adapting CHEP from CAHE and in evaluating the former, based on designs, measures, procedures and analysis adopted.

2.2 Study phase 1

2.2.1 Information gathering (stage one)

2.2.1.1 Design and participants

In the *formative phase* (July to September 2010) we collected data for development of CHEP by interviewing 40 purposively selected hypertensive patients using a modified version of the *interview guide* previously used for CAHE patients in the Netherlands [12, 24]. The interview guide was however tailored to the Nigerian context to make it culturally relevant for the priority patients of this study. We additionally searched available literature for relevant information on hypertension care and self-management in rural contexts. Using grounded theory we transcribed and analyzed the interviews each lasting about 90 minutes, for thematic contents simultaneously as they were conducted. The CAHE participants are mostly literate African immigrants in the Netherlands while most participants in CHEP are relatively illiterate native Africans from rural Nigeria. Furthermore, to increase cultural content of CHEP relative to CAHE, while CAHE used non-native Dutch nurse practitioners to collect data in English language, CHEP used native nurse and medical practitioners from the study region to collect data in familiar local languages (Yoruba and Nupe).

2.2.1.2 Measures

Beyond what was already known from CAHE, CHEP specifically sought to know the local, cultural and contextual factors the Nigerian hypertensive patients perceive as inhibitors or enablers of prescribed hypertension care and self-management: what hypertension is and how it presents; what situations make hypertension easy or difficult for patients to manage as advised; how patients' finances affect their treatment goals; and how patients' native customs and social environment affect their use of medications, food selection, exercise or weight management. During a follow-up focused group discussion (FGD) after CHEP counseling sessions, participants were further asked: how they view CHEP counseling on pills use, healthy diet, salt reduction/substitution and exercise; what was particularly helpful, or frustrating about CHEP counseling; how much they have been able to meet their hypertension self-management goals; and ways in which the education program can be improved upon in future.

2.2.1.3 Procedures

In addition to the qualitative interviews, at a later stage we conducted FGD with participants to get their views about usefulness, acceptability, sustainability and effectiveness or otherwise of CHEP. As was done in CAHE, the CHEP development interviews began with the interviewer familiarizing with respondents to determine preferred language of communication. Thereafter we introduced participants to the research objectives: to elicit patients' explanatory model of hypertension regarding cause, presentation, course, duration, consequence, treatment, self-management and contextual factors relating to hypertension including social, cultural, religious, and financial factors. Furthermore, while CAHE sought to know the effect migration had on hypertension self-management efforts of its immigrant participants, CHEP explored how peculiar local features of Nigeria's rural, social and cultural environments can be exploited to optimize hypertension self-care.

2.2.1.4 Analysis

We used MAXQDA data management software [29], and Grounded Theory [30] to analyze our data. The analytic process was at first carried out by two researchers independently, thereafter the interview transcripts were exchanged and coding and analytic steps repeated all over by individual researcher. Following this, areas of disagreement were jointly resolved by discussing the data further. In analyzing, we repeatedly examined, compared, verified and reordered the data in line with identified themes and concepts. This produced a matrix of concepts, sub-categories and categories from multi-level coding along thematic lines as follows: a) first we identified clusters of similar concepts in each interview transcript by assigning series of open codes to similar text fragments and emerging themes that reflected same ideas. To produce a code list we inductively coded sections of each transcript that provided information on respondents' ideas about hypertension and hypertension self-management; b) next we reviewed the code list to eliminate duplicates and streamline similar concepts to produce a smaller set of mutually exclusive concepts; and c) we scrutinized the data further and grouped streamlined concepts and related text fragments under four major themes to address our core research question: what social, cultural or native factors affect compliance with prescribed pills, diet and healthy behavior among hypertensive primary care patients from rural Nigeria?

2.2.2 Preliminary adaptation design (stage two)

In the preliminary adaptation stage, we tailored CHEP culturally using information collected in the *Information Gathering Stage*. Our underlying objective was to increase cultural content of CHEP. We made both *surface structure* and *deep structure* changes to the original contents of CHEP and CAHE to achieve a culturally adapted CHEP. *Surface Structure changes* refer to matching of educational intervention materials and messages to observable superficial characteristics of our target population e.g. use of familiar people, places, language, food, locations, and cultural activities preferred by the Nigerian patients, while *Deep Structure changes* involved incorporating social, cultural, environmental and historical components to influence the targeted hypertension self-management behavior among the Nigerian patients [7].

2.2.2.1 Design and participants

Both CHEP and CAHE had notable similarities in forms and contents; each was implemented in three modules over 6 months among hypertensive patients in Europe (*CAHE*), and Africa (*CHEP*). But there were differences in their designs. CAHE used non-native nurse practitioners as educators in English language, while CHEP used native medical doctor and nurse to deliver the educational intervention in local languages. Furthermore, while CAHE recruited participants from four primary care clinics in urban Amsterdam, CHEP recruited participants from a single primary care clinic in rural Nigeria. Unlike CHEP, patients in CAHE benefited from modern lifestyle referral support e.g. gyms in Amsterdam city in addition to exposure to a hypertension handbook. In contrast, patients in CHEP had exposure to educational materials that were contextually tailored to Nigerian rural context e.g. audiovisuals and poster teachings on dietary salt replacement with suitable local substitute *Iru*, and use of household chores, farming, fishing, gardening, leisure activities (drumming, gaming, dancing, singing) etc., as forms of exercise. The audiovisuals were scripted and acted by familiar faces including some participants themselves.

2.2.2.2 Measures

Excluding goals setting and few self-report measures, many other measures were assessed in both CAHE and CHEP including patient demographics and physiological measures. Other measures include perceived stress, social support, and illness perception, beliefs about medicines, self efficacy, medication adherence, lifestyle adherence and satisfaction with care. Unlike CHEP however, a measure of 'discrimination' was deemed relevant and included in CAHE whose participants had migrated to Europe and could possibly experience social exclusion.

2.2.2.3 Procedure

A CHEP counseling visit usually began with participants familiarizing with others and the trainers. This is followed by: group interactive counseling on hypertension and hypertension self-management; poster teaching on culturally relevant exercises; a visit to the local market to familiarize with healthy foods; an audiovisual viewing session on pills use, healthy diet and lifestyle; a field practical exercise session; and a goal setting and assessment session. CAHE on the other hand was delivered in one-on-one teaching sessions, featured no audiovisual session, and did not involve teaching visits to local market or grocery store but nevertheless deployed a specially prepared take-home hypertension handbook to teach her relatively more literate participants about healthy food choices, food preparation methods, pills use and healthy lifestyle. Both CAHE and CHEP counseling trainings were structured into 3 modules and delivered on 3 occasions few weeks apart, over six months in between a baseline and a final assessment visit. In both programs, every participant had physiological, anthropometric and self-report measurements at baseline and final visits. However, CHEP additionally had these measures taken during each of the 3 intervening educational visits because it was observed during pre-baseline information visits that the patients valued such interim measurements if the results are immediately communicated to motivate their self-management efforts.

2.3 *Study phase 2*

2.3.1 Preliminary adaptation testing (stage three)

2.3.1.1 Design and participants

The *preliminary adaptation testing* took place in the second phase of the study (March to August 2012) during which we used quasi-experimental pretest-posttest design to assess cultural fitness and effectiveness of the newly adapted CHEP. We included, trained and evaluated a cohort of 149 patients over a period of 6 months. Participants were evaluated on performance of set behavioral goals to assess cultural fitness. At a later stage we conducted an FGD with a sub-set of the participants to assess their perceptions about usefulness and acceptability of the adapted intervention.

2.3.1.2 Measures

We measured and recorded participants' socio-demographic parameters (age, gender, ethnicity, marital status, income level, employment status, educational status, alcohol use and tobacco use) and assessed their hypertension treatment outcomes including blood pressure control, body mass index, medication adherence, behavioral adherence as well as social support, satisfaction with care, illness perception, beliefs about medicines, and medication adherence self efficacy. Furthermore we asked participants specific questions on physical activity and exercise, use of salt, alcohol and smoking and graded their responses on a Likert Scale. Finally we asked participants to set and practice preferred culturally adapted behavioral health goals and graded their performances of set goals as a measure of 'cultural fitness.

2.3.1.3 Procedures

Each of the 149 participants individually had an initial baseline assessment, followed by 3 modules of CHEP training in groups of 12–15 at 6 weeks, 10 weeks and 14 weeks past baseline. They were later disaggregated to have final individual assessments at 6 months past baseline. In essence, each participant had five study visits including a baseline assessment visit, a final assessment visit and three intervening group educational and goals setting assessment visits. Following the baseline visit (1st study visit) each participant was guided to set 3 culturally adapted behavioral goals during the first training session (2nd study visit), and to practice the selected goals at home until he/she revisits for the second training session (3rd study visit). The same goals setting instructions were repeated at the end of second training towards the third and final training session (4th study visit). Participants were additionally guided to practice preferred physical exercises for 20 minutes during the 3rd training session only, and they were encouraged to continue the exercises at home until the final visits at 6 months (5th study visit). In the section on assessment of set goals, participants' goals related performances were rated on a Likert scale and compared over 6 months before and after the intervention. Full details of the effectiveness of CHEP evaluation study are available in a related study [13].

2.3.1.4 Analysis

Data were analyzed based on: 1) qualitative self-report from each of the 149 participants on performance of set goals as instructed; and 2) quantitative 'before-, and after' comparison of changes in treatment outcomes of participants following intervention.

In assessing performance of set goals, we recorded the number and types of goals set by each participant during a current visit following practice of such goals at home as instructed during previous visit. Using a Likert scale we inquired and got qualitative responses from each participant on the extent to which they practiced selected goals at home. For the CHEP effectiveness study we employed descriptive statistics and regression analysis to evaluate changes in BP control, Body Mass Index, behavioral adherence and medication adherence and got promising improvements as reported in Odusola, et al. [13].

Adaptation Refinement (Stage 4) and Cultural Adaptation Trial (Stage 5).

By design we have reserved the last two stages of the cultural adaptation process, '*Adaptation Refinement*' and '*Cultural Adaptation Trial*' for the near future to implement CHEP Efficacy Trial. This is similar to procedures adopted in a previous US study on cultural adaptation of an evidence based treatment, the MLP for Latinas sub-cultural group [11].

2.3.1.5 Ethics

Approval for Ethical conduct of the main study was obtained from the Ethics Committee of University of Ilorin Teaching Hospital on 30th March 2010. The current study is one of the sub-studies of the main study.

3. Results

We collected qualitative information from 40 hypertensive patients (systolic BP $\geq$ 140 mmHg and/or diastolic BP $\geq$ 90 mmHg). Most of them were 50 years or older, two third were Christians, almost all (80%) earn less than 5USD per day while 70% had only primary school education, and most were artisans engaged in farming, fishing, or petty trading (**Table 1**).

Characteristics	N (%)
Age group (years)	
• 30–50	9 (22.5%)
• 50–70	26 (65%)
• 70–90	5 (12.5%)
Gender	
• Male	16 (40%)
• Female	24 (60%)
Educational level	
• None or primary education	28 (70%)

Characteristics	N (%)
• Secondary education	9 (22.5%)
• Tertiary education	3 (7.5%)
Ethnicity	
• Nupe	6 (15%)
• Yoruba	31 (77.5%)
• Others	3 (7.5%)

Table 1.
Socio-demographic characteristics of participants.

Hereunder we describe our results based on the first three out of five guideline-based cultural adaptation stages.

3.1 *Information gathering (stage 1)*

The results are in two streams: a) *the cultural factors inhibiting uptake and practice of healthy behavior*; and b) *the cultural factors enabling uptake and practice of healthy behavior*.

A. **Cultural Inhibitors of Uptake and Practice of Healthy Behavior**

Our data showed that a people's culture, customs and beliefs have capacity to discourage uptake and practice of healthy behavior (**Table 2**).

1. **Increasing use of dietary salt**: certain cultural practices increase use of salt by the local population. During food preservation practices, salt is used to preserve fish and meat against microbial decomposition. For example, when asked about the cultural practices influencing salt use, a 56 year old hypertensive female [ID37] replied "*we normally preserve our meat from getting rotten by salting and drying them in the sun daily*". Food preparation practices also encourage increased use of salt. Some people have the habit of preparing meals with salt and salt-containing condiments e.g. maggi (salt *plus* hydrogenated oil *plus* monosodium glutamate). Others are accustomed to salty meals and would habitually add extra table salt to meals already prepared with salt. Some use the salty supernatant obtained from boiled meat to prepare soups believing this enhances its flavor. Furthermore, medicinal use of salt is common in the study region as it is common local practice to manage stomach upsets and abdominal discomforts by drinking salted water (salt solution).

2. **Increasing body weight and size**: some cultural practices encourage weight gain. A large body size is a desirable appearance to some as societal sign of affluence, comfort or wealth. And so, people may embark on intentional weight gain merely to show off perceived wealth or affluence. Furthermore, it is often perceived that a large body size enhances a woman's beauty or sexual attractiveness. There is societal perception that the fatter a lady is the more beautiful and fresh she is. On weight gain, a 50 year old female, [ID3] responded: "*people often see being fat as synonymous with affluence, comfort and peace of mind, and they sometimes associate robustness with beauty in women. Moreover, some of us women prefer to get fat believing that by so doing we are more attractive to our husbands and to men generally.* Our data further shows that people can

sometimes get discouraged when exercising to lose weight For example, an elderly male respondent [ID30] clarified a question on weight reduction saying *"in this region, people often link slimming down to disease particularly if the weight loss is pronounced, suggesting such might be due to disease,* and that *"slim people are miserly and would rather not spend enough money to feed well and get big".*

3. **Physical inactivity and lack of exercise**: excerpts from our data show there is a strong cultural correlation between societal perception and 'need or needlessness' to exercise. Many believe exercise is a needless waste of time. Some perceive exercise as dangerous to health especially with advancing age when the body is assumed fragile and weaker. Deliberate attempts to exercise by trekking to destinations are perceived negatively. Such persons are taunted as being miserly and reluctant to fund transport costs to their destinations. On challenges encountered in exercising, an elderly male [ID30] said *"when people see me walking 'to exercise' they often slight me and make derogatory comments that I'm greedy and would rather walk long distances than spend money on transportation.*

4. **Use of tobacco and other stimulants**: curiously, social habits like use of stimulants and tobacco products are sometimes perceived as promoting health. A popular local alcoholic brew '*Palm wine*' is believed to make vision clearer while others like the '*Ogogoro*' (local gin), *Snuff* (Nicotine powder) and *Taba (fine-ground tobacco leaves)* are variously perceived to relieve stress and bodily tension, and stimulate work. Now better informed, a 65 year old male [ID23] regretted: *"our fore fathers used to say palm wine makes one see very well, but it is now glaring to me that such views were misplaced.* Another participant [ID29] responded: *"in this region we believe chewing kola nuts and using snuff stimulate performance of household chores and work although I personally don't use them".*

B. **Cultural Facilitators of Uptake and Practice of Healthy Behavior**

Our data yielded a rich mix of information on factors encouraging healthy behavior among participants (**Table 2**). Many felt cultural adaptation of certain local practices made it easier, cheaper and more attractive to practice healthy behavior.

Category	Sub-category		Concepts and Examples
	Factors motivating healthy behavior	**Factors inhibiting healthy behavior**	
Food related practices: Salt use		Food conservation practices	Salt can preserve food stocks against microbial degradation [n = 3]*
		Food preparation practices	A salt-less diet is repulsive to the African mindset [n = 7]
			Salt and salt products (e.g. maggi) are substantially used in meals preparation [n = 14]
		Medicinal use of salt	Salted water (salt solution) is a sure panacea for abdominal/ stomach discomfort [n = 3]

Category	Sub-category		Concepts and Examples
	Factors motivating healthy behavior	**Factors inhibiting healthy behavior**	
Food related practices: Salt use	Availability of suitable salt substitute ***Iru***		Following health counseling, I found out that meals prepared with *Iru* in place of salt are tastier and more delicious [n = 2]
Food related practices: Fruits and vegetables consumption	Endowment of rural environments with health-promoting possibilities and practices: arable land for vegetable and fruit farming and poultry; and streams and rivers for fishing		I now get enough vegetables in my regular diet from vegetable gardening at my backyard [n = 5]
Societal socio-cultural perceptions: weight gain		Increase in body size perceived as wealth, affluence, comfort	The bigger one is the wealthier, affluent and more comfortable he/she is perceived [n = 12]
		Decrease in body size perceived as illness, disease	Deliberate weight loss or slimming down perceived as being caused by serious internal disease [n = 13]
		Increase in body size (bigness) perceived as a woman's beauty or sexual attractiveness	The fatter a woman is, the more beautiful and attractive she is viewed [n = 7]
		Weight gain or Obesity perceived inherited or natural in some families	Heaviness or fatness runs in my family; we normally have big sizes [n = 3]
		Some local delicacies have fattening tendency	Popular local meals are often heavily starch-based, e.g. Pounded yam, Garri-eba [n = 5]
			Red Palm-oil, Groundnut oil readily available in our environment [n = 11]
			Popular local goat-breeding practice makes red meat readily available [n = 2]
Socio-cultural perceptions: weight reduction	Cultural perceptions and orientations: being fat is tantamount to ugliness, sluggishness and physical unfitness		People will say: look at him, 'big for nothing', he will not be able to enjoy breathing, worse still [n = 3].
Socio-cultural perceptions: lack of exercise		Perception of exercise as related to elderly "fragile" health and wellbeing	Popular view: exercising is dangerous with increasing age, and to health the elderly [n = 7]
		Perception of exercise as related to perceived necessity	Popular view: walking long distances just to exercise could only mean one is unserious and greedy to avoid spending travel costs [n = 5]

Category	Sub-category		Concepts and Examples
	Factors motivating healthy behavior	**Factors inhibiting healthy behavior**	
Socio-cultural perceptions: exercise and physical fitness	Cultural practices and environmental possibilities to achieve physical fitness		Brisk trekking to farm, other destinations; dancing and clapping in church; drumming during festivals; food grains grinding and yam pounding; farming and gardening activities; laundry (washing clothes), sweeping floors,; and where feasible canoe paddling on rivers
Socio-cultural perceptions: social habits		Smoking and non-smoking tobacco and Snuff uses are wrongly perceived beneficial to health	Cigarette smoking and Snuff sniffing relieve tension and aid work [n = 1]
		There's a perception that local alcoholic beverage (Palm wine) and Kola nuts are beneficial to health	Palm wine makes vision clearer [n = 1], chewing kola nuts stimulate task performance and it's a social standard for elders to chew kola nuts [n = 2]
Socio-cultural perceptions: social habits	Faith-based and gender-based considerations that discourages use of alcohol and tobacco		Faith-based and gender-based abhorrence of smoking, alcohol and tobacco by women; society frowns seriously at sight of a woman smoking cigarette

Notes: n refers to the number of respondents who expressed the implied view.

Table 2.
Motivational and inhibitory factors of healthy behavior: Thematic matrix of categories, sub-categories and concepts.

1. **Limiting use of dietary salt**: following enlightenment through the adapted education program some participants realized that *Iru* (a local food condiment) is a suitable and effective alternative to dietary salt. *Iru,* the locally grown African Locust Bean seed is a relatively cheaper food condiment commonly available. It is devoid of salt or sodium derivatives and participants agreed it makes food tastier and more delicious. Many now use *Iru* in place of salt to prepare their meals although few confessed they nonetheless add little salt despite using Iru. A 50 year old female [ID11] said "*I have been enlightened and I have since been using Iru in place of salt to prepare my family meals; truly I found out the meals so prepared are tastier and more delicious.*

2. **Increasing consumption of dietary fruits and vegetables**: our data shows that rural African communities are endowed with potential for promoting health using existing socio-cultural and environmental peculiarities such as arable lands, domesticated animals and flourishing streams and rivers. They provide opportunities for vegetable farming, fishing, poultry and animal husbandry. To some participants, earning a living through these *health-related* economic activities motivate hypertension self-management efforts. When asked how often he consumes fruits and vegetables an elderly participant [ID32] responded: "*based on advice from my doctor, I now practice vegetable farming on the*

large expanse of land at my backyard which before now had laid waste, and from this I get sufficient supply of vegetables to meet my family needs".

3. **Decreasing body size and weight**: some female participants perceive cultural linkages between health and body size, health and wealth, and health and beauty. In the study region, there was a popular cultural perception that "the fatter a woman is the more affluent, comfortable or beautiful she is". This perception has health implications as it encourages undue weight gain among the women. However, this perception is changing nowadays, and being too fat is now viewed as ugliness, sluggishness or physical unfitness. When asked what relationship exists between beauty and large body sizes, a respondent [ID26] replied: "*beauty is a good thing that sometimes goes with bigness but some people are ugly looking when fat*". These newer perceptions have helped many to adopt healthier behavior.

4. **Increasing physical activity and exercise**: although some participants view exercise as dangerous to health because of advancing age, many others nonetheless understood that exercise is generally good for health and helps to control their hypertension. After the educational counseling many are now aware that some level of physical fitness can be achieved using usual everyday activities in rural communities, and that exercising do not necessarily require formal regimented sessions like street jogging, gyms and swimming pools sessions applicable to cities and urban towns. Our data showed that if given relevant encouragement and training, participants are able and willing to adopt culturally modified versions of local practices to achieve physical fitness: *walking briskly and regularly to farm and other destinations; faith-based and cultural dancing, drumming, clapping or singing; food preparation practices like pounding yam and grains in mortars; farming and gardening activities including shoveling and hoeing; traditional laundry (washing clothes), sweeping floors, and drawing or fetching water from wells; and where feasible canoe paddling on rivers and cycling to move around*. A participant [ID21] responded: "*in my community, women prepare the popular local delicacy pounded yam using mortar, this being a form of exercise since they sweat a lot when they pound*".

5. **Limiting use of alcohol, tobacco and stimulants**: some participants leverage on existing cultural and religious perceptions to acquire healthy behavior. Following behavioral counseling the few who use tobacco (smoking and non-smoking forms) were able to exploit existing *gender-based,* and *faith-based cultural perceptions* to discontinue such practices, including faith-based religious abhorrence of smoking and use of alcohol, and gender-based disapproval of female use of tobacco, alcohol, and snuff. It is culturally reprehensible to see a woman smoking cigarette in rural communities.

3.2 Preliminary adaptation design (stage two)

Cultural adaptation of the Education Program was accomplished based on the conceptual framework of formative research using information obtained from qualitative interviews with patients. The other anticipated source of information, literature review, did not yield much useful information on the topic from the study region. Osuna et al. similarly relied substantially on information from a Focus Group Discussion with participants to achieve cultural adaptation design of a diabetes Intervention program among Latinas in the United States [11]. The adaptation in our study was achieved through cultural modification of existing behavioral health practices among the local population. This involved modifying the *'form'* (surface structure elements) and the *'specific content'* (deep structure elements) into culturally friendly and adoptable methods of exercising within rural contexts. However, because information from our interviews also revealed local practices and beliefs perceived inhibitory to healthy behavior, we highlighted and discarded the inhibitory perceptions in order to achieve a culturally attractive and acceptable final behavioral counseling program. **Table 3** displays a synopsis of key differences and similarities in contents and procedures between the culturally adapted program (CHEP) and the adaptable program (CAHE).

Program Content & Procedure	CAHE	CHEP
Type of program	Hypertension education program	Hypertension education program
Focus of program	Hypertension self-management	Hypertension self-management
Implementation setting	Urban Amsterdam, Netherlands	Rural Kwara, Nigeria
Study population	Hypertensive Primary care African immigrants (mostly literate)	Hypertensive primary care native Africans (mostly illiterate)
Language of communication	English	Native Yoruba and Nupe
Cultural familiarity of education counselors or trainers	Used Dutch nurse Practitioner	Used native African medical and nurse practitioners
Information gathering method	Qualitative interviews with hypertensive participants	FGD and Qualitative interviews with hypertensive participants
Cultural exploratory content	Exploratory from a perspective of European urban/city environment	More deeply exploratory from a perspective of rural African socio-cultural environment
Behavioral health facilities available to support physical fitness and exercise habits	Promoted use of lifestyle referral facilities like gyms, swimming pool, walking out etc.	Promoted use of cultural and environmental possibilities like household chores, farm work, food preparation activities etc.
Adapted component of dietary counseling	Counseled participants to reduce dietary salt consumption	Supported dietary salt reduction counseling with possibility to replace salt with a suitable local substitute *Iru*
Assessment of cultural fitness	Did not assess participants for cultural fitness	Assessed participants for cultural fitness using culturally tailored behavioral health goals
Effect on hypertension treatment outcome	Significant improvements in diastolic blood pressure and lifestyle adherence	Significant improvements in blood pressure control, medication adherence and lifestyle adherence

Notes: CAHE – Culturally appropriate hypertension education; CHEP – Cardiovascular health education program.

Table 3.
Contents and procedural variances and similarities between culturally adapted CHEP and CAHE.

Furthermore, in **Table 4** we highlight the thematic categories of the relationships existing between traditional local perspectives and cultural practices, and their adaptability following educational counseling drawing from newly available culturally relevant information.

Category	Sub-category	Cultural perspectives and linkages	Cultural adaptation and tailoring
Cultural endowments towards healthy behavior – Diet	Rural African food preservation and preparation practices	Africans are naturally accustomed to high-salt diet	Ability to replace salt with Iru, a suitable local substitute
	Medicinal use of salt	Health-driven ignorant use of salt further diminishes health	Provide enlightenment information about avoidable use of salt
Cultural awareness towards healthy behavior – Weight	Local perceptions about body image and size	Societal perception driven preference for big body sizes	Provide useful information to situate body size within health perspectives
Cultural re-orientation towards healthy behavior – Exercise	Perceived danger of exercise to health	Health-driven concerns about older age-related dangers of exercise	Re-orientate about benefits/risks of age-tailored exercising
Cultural practices and environmental endowments towards healthy behavior – Physical activity	Perceptions that it is difficult, expensive and time wasting to achieve physical fitness	Realizations that physical fitness is also achievable using usual everyday household chores, cultural and occupational activities, leisure and faith-based activities	Re-orientate patients about the possibility and practicability of cheap, user-friendly, attractive and acceptable cultural and environmental activities as exercise
Faith-based and societal perspectives and norms	Societal perceptions of certain behaviors as 'unfaithful' and 'anti-social' e.g. smoking and use of alcohol	Health-driven exploitation of faith-based abhorrence of certain norms to drive healthy behavior	Provide useful information to exploit faith-based and gender-based socio-cultural practices

Table 4.
Culturally adapted components of existing behavioral practices: Categories, sub-categories, concepts and thematic linkages.

3.3 Preliminary adaptation testing (stage 3)

Preliminary evaluation of the culturally adapted educational intervention was implemented in two arms: 1) cultural fitness assessment based on performance of set behavioral health goals; and 2) assessment of effectiveness based on changes in participants' hypertension treatment outcomes.

To assess cultural fitness, we examined and recorded serial performance of set goals as reported by participants themselves over six 6 months.

Simultaneously, the effectiveness assessment study took place over same period but this not being the focus of the current study, is reported fully elsewhere [13]. Briefly it involved before-, and after assessments of changes in blood pressure (BP) control, medication adherence, behavioral adherence, and body mass index (BMI). Out of an initial 149 included participants, 140 (94%) completed the study. More participants reported high adherence to prescribed medications and behavioral advice at 6 months compared to baseline: respectively, 101 (72%) at 6 months versus 70 (50%) at baseline, ($p < 0.001$) and 126 (90%) at 6 months versus 106 (76%) at baseline, ($p < 0.001$). Similarly, participants with controlled BP doubled from 34 (24%) at baseline to 65 (46%) at 6 months, ($p = 0.001$). The median SBP and DBP decreased from 129.0 to 122.0 mmHg, ($p = 0.002$) and from 80.0 to 73.5 mmHg, ($p < 0.001$), respectively. However, BMI did not change ($p = 0.444$). The improvement in medication adherence was associated with a decrease in medication concerns ($p = 0.045$) and improvement in medication self-efficacy ($p < 0.001$).

3.3.1 Performance assessment of set goals

As indicated in the methods each participant made 5 visits over 6 months: a baseline assessment visit, three intervening group education visits, and a final assessment visit. Hereunder we report the performance of set goals by participants based on self-reports. Using information from our interview data we structured existing local behavioral health practices of the region into 12 distinct culturally tailored goals (**Box 1**). We guided participants to select, set and practice three preferred goals during the three intervening group visits as well as at home in the weeks that followed their current visit. Their performances were assessed qualitatively during the subsequent visits.

We inquired verbally from participants about how well they practiced selected goals during a subsequent visit and graded their responses on a Likert scale as follows:

1. To reduce amount of salt and salt-containing condiments I currently use in food preparation and/ or preservation by half before my next visit
2. To completely replace salt with *Iru* in all my food preparation and food preservation processes before my next visit
3. To increase my consumption of healthy foods by eating more fish and at least 3 servings of vegetables and fruits daily before my next visit
4. To decrease my consumption of unhealthy foods by eating less of red palm oil, groundnut oil, goat meat and other fatty food daily before my next visit
5. To stop smoking completely if I do, or at least reduce the number of cigarette sticks I smoke daily by half before my next visit
6. To completely discontinue the use of all socially acceptable non-smoking forms of tobacco (Taba/Snuff), and Kola nuts, or reduce the quantity I use daily by half before my next visit
7. To completely discontinue consumption of Alcohol and other alcoholic beverages (Spirit, Palm wine, Gin, Ogogoro) perceived as culturally acceptable, or at least reduce the quantities I consume daily by half before my next visit
8. To exercise more regularly using locally available methods like brisk walking, canoe paddling, cycling or others, to and from my destinations for at least 30 minutes everyday
9. To exercise more regularly using food preparation processes such as yam/grain pounding in mortars whenever feasible over at least 30 minutes per session before my next visit
10. To exercise more regularly using usual household chores such as sweeping floors, laundry (washing clothes), pulling/fetching water from wells or others over at least 30 minutes daily before my next visit
11. To exercise more regularly using usual farming activities such as ground hoeing, shoveling, bush clearing, manual harvesting, gardening etc. over at least 30 minutes daily before my next visit
12. To exercise more regularly using usual leisurely or faith-related activities such as clapping, dancing, singing, drumming, gaming or others for at least 30 minutes daily before my next visit

Box 1.
Culturally tailored behavioral health goals set by participants

DOI: http://dx.doi.org/10.5772/intechopen.94542

1. For how many days in a week did you perform the selected goal?

   Response grading: 0-1 day (poor); 2–3 days (fair); 4–5 days (good); 6–7 days (very good)

2. For how many minutes in a day did you perform the selected goal?

   Response grading: 0–10 mins (poor); 11–20 mins (fair); 21–30 mins (good); > 30 mins (very good)

3. How seriously did you perceive any challenges or difficulties encountered in performing the goals you selected and how well did you resolve the challenges?

   Response grading: serious challenges, not resolved (poor); moderate challenges, partly resolved (fair); minor challenges, fully resolved (good); encountered no challenges (very good)

4. On a scale of 1 to 4 (1 – poor, 2 – fair, 3 – good, 4 – very good), how would you rate yourself on degree of performance (effectiveness), of set goals?

   Response: not performed at all (poor); sometimes performed (fair); often performed (good); always performed (very good).

Following this we graded self-rated performances of participants on a Likert scale (**Table 5**), and found that an overwhelming majority of them performed the selected goals reasonably well. At least 49% and 28% of participants were graded 'good' and 'very good' respectively on the number of minutes they performed selected goals daily. Furthermore, regarding number of days per week they performed selected goals, about 61% and 11% were graded 'good' and 'very good' respectively. On their abilities to resolve potential challenges faced, 18% and 56% of participants were graded 'good' and 'very good' respectively. Finally 30% and 53% of participants were graded 'good' and 'very good' respectively regarding their perceived effectiveness in performing selected goals.

Performance scale	Participants' graded performance (Minutes/day)	Participants' graded performance (Days/week)	Participants' graded performance (Resolution of challenges)	Participants' self-rated goals performance (Effectiveness)
	N (%)	N (%)	N (%)	N (%)
Poor	23 (16)	21 (15)	11 (8)	0
Fair	10 (7)	19 (14)	25 (18)	24 (17)
Good	68 (49)	85 (61)	25 (18)	42 (30)
Very good	39 (28)	15 (11)	79 (56)	74 (53)
Total	140 (100)	140 (100)	140 (100)	140 (100)

Table 5.
Assessment of performance of set goals by participants.

3.3.2 Preferential practice of particular behavioral goals

The particular types of culturally adapted goals participants preferred to set and pursue yielded interesting information from our data. Viewed against the background of attractiveness and acceptability, such information can be useful in guiding physicians and care givers on behavioral health practices likely to be accepted and complied with by hypertensive patients. This type of information can predict areas in need of counseling reinforcement for patients in efforts to improve hypertension self-management skills. Extracts from our data (**Table 6**) reveals that the three most preferred and set goals are dietary salt reduction, exercising and compliance with pills use. Similarly, the three least preferred and set goals are stopping tobacco use, limiting alcohol use and stopping kola nuts consumption. Finally, important considerations that guided participants in selecting particular goals include funding performance of the goals, ease/rigor of performance, and access to practicing the goals.

Types of Goals	**Educational Sessions**		
	CHEP 1, N (%)	**CHEP 2, N (%)**	**CHEP 3, N (%)**
Diet (salt restriction)	124 (89)	97 (69)	66 (47)
Diet (fat restriction)	23 (16)	12 (9)	27 (19)
Diet (vegetables & fruits consumption)	16 (11)	9 (6)	8 (6)
Physical fitness & exercise	121 (86)	100 (71)	93 (66)
Weight reduction	59 (42)	47 (34)	32 (23)
Quit smoking	4 (3)	4 (3)	2 (1)
Quit non-smoked tobacco	5 (4)	2 (1)	0 (0)
Quit Kola nut	14 (10)	4 (3)	7 (5)
Restrict alcohol	13 (9)	10 (7)	7 (5)
Comply with pills use	92 (66)	78 (56)	59 (42)
Comply with clinic appointments	13 (9)	19 (14)	15 (11)

Table 6.
Frequency and types of behavioral goals set during educational sessions.

4. Discussion

We examined the proceedings and results of cultural adaptation of a behavioral treatment program following standard guidelines, among primary care patients with hypertension from rural Nigeria highlighting cultural fitness and effectiveness of the adapted program on their hypertension self-management. Based on theoretical and conceptual framework of formative research described by Resnicow et al. [7], we combined information from exploratory interviews with hypertensive patients with extracts from a review of literature on the topic to adapt a Cardiovascular Health Education Program (CHEP) from an existing Culturally Appropriate Hypertension Education (CAHE) previously deployed among hypertensive African immigrants in the Netherlands [12]. The literature review however did not yield enough relevant information. Our goal was to increase cultural sensitivity and contents of CHEP relative to CAHE and to make the adapted CHEP relevant to specific needs of hypertensive patients from rural Nigeria. Resnicow et al. had proposed combining: a) *surface structure elements* (matching of adaptable behavioral practices and materials to observable superficial characteristics of the target population); with b) *deep structure elements* (incorporation of target population's customs, culture, beliefs and values into their existing adaptable practices). Drawing inspirations from this, CHEP used materials from both *surface structures* and *deep structures* in its development and adaptation processes. We additionally followed the guidelines described by Barrera et al. in a consensus of cultural adaption processes [10] in adapting CHEP. Finally we evaluated the adapted program and found that CHEP improved participants' hypertension treatment outcomes and enabled increased performance of culturally tailored behavioral health goals among the participants.

Cultural adaptation is the systematic modification of an existing evidence-based treatment to conform with a distinct group's language, culture, customs and local cultural contexts in a way that it becomes compatible with the group's cultural orientations and values" [9]. The cultural modification process enhances attractiveness and adoptability of a new program among targeted populations. The promising results reported in the previous CHEP evaluation study [13], are plausible in the light of findings from other studies in support of views that standardized cultural adaptation of behavioral interventions can improve treatment outcomes [9, 14, 15, 21, 31]. To the best of our knowledge no previous study conducted in rural African context has shown such potentials from implementing culturally adapted interventions.

Following debates on the most appropriate process for cultural adaptation, researchers arrived at a consensus aggregating various approaches to establish a standard guideline involving five sequential stages: 1) information gathering, stage one; 2) preliminary adaptation design, stage two; 3) preliminary adaptation testing, stage three; 4) adaptation refinement, stage four; and 5) adaptation trial, stage five [10, 17]. In the current study however, by design we opted to adapt CHEP from CAHE using the first three of five guideline-based stages, deferring the last two stages for a future CHEP efficacy trial. A diabetes lifestyle intervention program was similarly adapted for Latinas in the USA using stages one to three only [11].

The local and cultural environments of patients in our study are endowed with materials and possibilities that influenced their hypertension self-management capacities. We found that locally grown Locust Beans '*Iru*' is a healthier condiment suitable in replacing dietary salt. This finding is strikingly comparable to a Peruvian study which reported successful introduction of a similar *salt substitute* with less elemental sodium among a local hypertensive population [32]. Our results also showed that exercising can be attractive and easier when performed using traditional household chores and cultural practices.

Cultural fitness is determined by the extent to which a people accept and use the language, values, beliefs and materials characteristics of newly introduced culturally tailored interventions targeting their self-management skills. We assessed the adapted intervention for cultural fitness by conducting a goals setting and performance exercise among participants and got promising results on performances by most participants. Similar findings have also been reported from other studies [19–21]. Moreover during a follow-up FGD participants spoke excitedly and expressed desires to continue to use the education program even after the study. Interestingly we observed that the three most common behavioral goals practiced by participants were *salt reduction, exercise and weight reduction* while the three least commonly practiced goals were *smoking cessation, alcohol reduction and cessation of kola nuts use*. We believe such observations reflect new perceptions of the health risks which participants now associate with the habits following enlightenment from behavioral counseling. Such information on preferred and disliked behavioral practices can help physicians make informed decisions on areas most in need of attention in planning behavioral health interventions for patients with cardiovascular risk factors.

Limitations encountered in this study include:

1. Participants could have been biased in recalling events and they may have given socially desirable answers on some aspects of our results that are based on self-reports

2. Without prejudice to results obtained, logistics and funding constraints limited our ability to implement all the five guideline-based cultural adaptation stages

5. Conclusion

We followed standard guidelines to culturally adapt an existing behavioral health intervention among hypertensive patients from rural Nigeria. Modeled after a similar intervention from Europe we systematically developed and adapted the new intervention using frameworks of formative research. We got quite promising results on evaluating the adapted intervention for cultural fitness and effectiveness. We submit that guide-line based culturally adapted behavioral treatments have potential to improve hypertension treatment outcomes and limit cardiovascular diseases.

5.1 Implication for practice

The successful control of risk factors among patients at risk of cardiovascular diseases is a major goal of every attending physician. But a major obstacle to this goal is the difficulties faced by patients in adhering to prescribed pills and behavioral advices. Innovations like the current intervention which provides unique information on behavioral practices preferred and disliked by patients can guide physicians on acceptable and adoptable behaviors.

Acknowledgements

Authors are grateful to the staff of Ogo Oluwa hospital and the health insurance company. We thank Health Insurance Fund, PharmAccess Foundation, and NUFFIC for supporting the study.

Conflict of interest

The authors declare no conflict of interest.

Author contributions

AO drafted the manuscript, designed and conducted the study. AA revised versions of the draft. Both authors approved the final draft.

Author details

Aina Olufemi Odusola[1*] and Ayoade Adedokun[2]

1 Department of Community Health and Primary Health Care, Lagos State University Teaching Hospital, Lagos, Nigeria

2 Department of Family Medicine, Lagos State University Teaching Hospital, Lagos, Nigeria

*Address all correspondence to: f.odusola@gmail.com

References

[1] Commodore-Mensah Y, Samuel LJ, Dennison-Himmelfarb CR, Agyemang C. Hypertension and overweight/obesity in Ghanaians and Nigerians living in West Africa and industrialized countries: a systematic review. J Hypertens. 2014 Mar;32(3): 464.

[2] Kengne AP, Awah PK, Fezeu L, Mbanya JC. The burden of high blood pressure and related risk factors in urban Sub-Saharan Africa: Evidences from Douala in Cameroon. Afr Health Sci [Internet]. 2007 Jan 1 [cited 2018 Mar 18];7(1). Available from: https://www.ajol.info/index.php/ahs/article/view/6989

[3] The top 10 causes of death [Internet]. [cited 2020 Feb 4]. Available from: https://www.who.int/news-room/fact-sheets/detail/the-top-10-causes-of-death

[4] Cardiovascular diseases [Internet]. [cited 2020 Feb 4]. Available from: https://www.who.int/westernpacific/health-topics/cardiovascular-diseases

[5] Hendriks ME, Wit FWNM, Roos MTL, Brewster LM, Akande TM, Beer IH de, et al. Hypertension in Sub-Saharan Africa: Cross-Sectional Surveys in Four Rural and Urban Communities. PLOS ONE. 2012 Mar 12;7(3):e32638.

[6] Ike SO, Aniebue PN, Aniebue UU. Knowledge, perceptions and practices of lifestyle-modification measures among adult hypertensives in Nigeria. Trans R Soc Trop Med Hyg. 2010 Jan 1;104(1): 55–60.

[7] Resnicow K, Baranowski T, Ahluwalia JS, Braithwaite RL. Cultural sensitivity in public health: defined and demystified. Ethn Dis. 1999;9(1):10–21.

[8] Netto G, Bhopal R, Lederle N, Khatoon J, Jackson-Morris A. How Can Health Promotion Interventions Be Adapted for Minority Ethnic Communities? Five Principles for Guiding the Development of Behavioural Interventions. Health Promot Int. 2010 Mar 1;25:248–57.

[9] Domenech Rodríguez MM, Baumann AA, Schwartz AL. Cultural Adaptation of an Evidence Based Intervention: From Theory to Practice in a Latino/a Community Context. Am J Community Psychol. 2011 Mar 1;47(1–2):170–86.

[10] Barrera M, Castro FG, Strycker LA, Toobert DJ. Cultural Adaptations of Behavioral Health Interventions: A Progress Report. J Consult Clin Psychol. 2013 Apr;81(2):196–205.

[11] Osuna D, Barrera M, Strycker LA, Toobert DJ, Glasgow RE, Geno CR, et al. Methods for the Cultural Adaptation of a Diabetes Lifestyle Intervention for Latinas: An Illustrative Project. Health Promot Pract. 2011 May 1;12(3):341–8.

[12] Beune EJAJ, Charante EPM van, Beem L, Mohrs J, Agyemang CO, Ogedegbe G, et al. Culturally Adapted Hypertension Education (CAHE) to Improve Blood Pressure Control and Treatment Adherence in Patients of African Origin with Uncontrolled Hypertension: Cluster-Randomized Trial. PLOS ONE. 2014 Mar 5;9(3): e90103.

[13] Odusola A, Nelissen H, Hendriks M, Schultsz C, Wit F, Bolarinwa O, et al. How Group-Based Cardiovascular Health Education Affects Treatment Adherence and Blood Pressure Control among Insured Hypertensive Nigerians: A Pre-Test, Post-Test Study. World J Cardiovasc Dis. 2015 Aug 1;5:181–98.

[14] Azizan A, Justine M, Kuan CS. Effects of a Behavioral Program on Exercise Adherence and Exercise

Self-Efficacy in Community-Dwelling Older Persons. Curr Gerontol Geriatr Res [Internet]. 2013 [cited 2018 Mar 10];2013. Available from: https://www.ncbi.nlm.nih.gov/pmc/articles/PMC3893800/

[15] Serour M, Alqhenaei H, Al-Saqabi S, Mustafa A-R, Ben-Nakhi A. Cultural factors and patients' adherence to lifestyle measures. Br J Gen Pr. 2007 Apr 1;57(537):291–5.

[16] Nierkens V, Hartman MA, Nicolaou M, Vissenberg C, Beune EJAJ, Hosper K, et al. Effectiveness of cultural adaptations of interventions aimed at smoking cessation, diet, and/or physical activity in ethnic minorities. a systematic review. PloS One. 2013;8(10):e73373.

[17] Castro FG, Barrera M, Holleran Steiker LK. Issues and Challenges in the Design of Culturally Adapted Evidence-Based Interventions. Annu Rev Clin Psychol. 2010;6(1):213–39.

[18] DeWalt DA, Davis TC, Wallace AS, Seligman HK, Bryant-Shilliday B, Arnold CL, et al. Goal setting in diabetes self-management: Taking the baby steps to success. Patient Educ Couns. 2009 Nov 1;77(2):218–23.

[19] Nothwehr F, Yang J. Goal setting frequency and the use of behavioral strategies related to diet and physical activity. Health Educ Res. 2007 Aug 1;22(4):532–8.

[20] Pearson ES. Goal setting as a health behavior change strategy in overweight and obese adults: A systematic literature review examining intervention components. Patient Educ Couns. 2012 Apr 1;87(1):32–42.

[21] Strecher VJ, Seijts GH, Kok GJ, Latham GP, Glasgow R, DeVellis B, et al. Goal Setting as a Strategy for Health Behavior Change. Health Educ Q. 1995 Jul;22(2):190–200.

[22] Odusola AO, Hendriks M, Schultsz C, Bolarinwa OA, Akande T, Osibogun A, et al. Perceptions of inhibitors and facilitators for adhering to hypertension treatment among insured patients in rural Nigeria: a qualitative study. BMC Health Serv Res. 2014 Dec 10;14(1):624.

[23] Olufemi Odusola A, Stronks K, Schultsz C, Hendriks M, Akeem Bolarinwa O, Akande T, et al. Development of cardiovascular health education program for primary care patients with hypertension in rural Nigeria: a qualitative study. Health Educ Care [Internet]. 2017 [cited 2020 Jul 30];2(1). Available from: http://oatext.com/Development-of-cardiovascular-health-education-program-for-primary-care-patients-with-hypertension-in-rural-Nigeria-a-qualitative-study.php

[24] Beune E. Culturally appropriate hypertension care: from patients' perspectives towards practical tools. 2010 Jan 1;

[25] Beune EJ, Haafkens JA, Agyemang C, Schuster JS, Willems DL. How Ghanaian, African-Surinamese and Dutch patients perceive and manage antihypertensive drug treatment: a qualitative study: J Hypertens. 2008 Apr;26(4):648–56.

[26] Odusola AO, Hendriks M, Schultsz C, Stronks K, Lange J, Osibogun A, et al. Development and evaluation of a patient centered cardiovascular health education program for insured patients in rural Nigeria (QUICK - II). BMC Public Health. 2011 Mar 21;11(1):171.

[27] Hendriks ME, Bolarinwa OA, Wit FWNW, Brewster LM, Odusola AO, Rosendaal NTA, et al. Feasibility and quality of cardiovascular disease prevention within a community-based health insurance program in rural Nigeria. J Hypertens. 33(2):366–75.

[28] Hygeia Community Health Plan (HCHP) | The Center for Health Market Innovations [Internet]. [cited 2020 Jul 28]. Available from: https://healthmarketinnovations.org/program/hygeia-community-health-plan-hchp

[29] Kuckartz DU. Udo Kuckartz Realizing Mixed-Methods Approaches with MAXQDA. :22.

[30] Corbin JM, Strauss A. Grounded theory research: Procedures, canons, and evaluative criteria. Qual Sociol. 1990 Mar 1;13(1):3–21.

[31] Heurtin-Roberts S, Reisin E. The Relation of Culturally Influenced Lay Models of Hypertension to Compliance With Treatment. Am J Hypertens. 1992 Nov 1;5(11):787–92.

[32] Pesantes MA, Diez-Canseco F, Bernabé-Ortiz A, Ponce-Lucero V, Miranda JJ. Taste, Salt Consumption, and Local Explanations around Hypertension in a Rural Population in Northern Peru. Nutrients [Internet]. 2017 Jul 5 [cited 2018 Mar 9];9(7). Available from: https://www.ncbi.nlm.nih.gov/pmc/articles/PMC5537813/

Chapter 5

Visual Disability and Causes of Preventable Blindness

Mercedes Libeth Ramos Amador
and Javier Eduardo Escober Torres

Abstract

The World Health Organization (WHO) estimates, worldwide, approximately 1300 million people with a form of visual impairment. More than 314 million have a severe visual impairment. Of these, 37 million are blind and 124 million suffer from low vision. Eighty percent of all these cases are considered avoidable. The main causes of blindness from one country to another, in order of frequency, are cataract (39%), uncorrected refractive errors (18%), and glaucoma (10%). In Latin America and the Caribbean, the loss of vision in adults continues to be a public health problem. Blindness and visual impairment tombs have a remarkable impact on the socioeconomic development of individuals and societies and the prevention of avoidable visual disabilities in the long term in terms of attention to health care and social expenditures. Of all the organs of the body, the eye is more accessible to direct examination. The visual function can be evaluated by means of simple subjective tests. The same can be taken care of from an adequate primary care service.

Keywords: blindness, cataract, refractive errors, glaucoma, visual acuity

1. Introduction

The universal aging of the population is a global concern because of its association with degenerative diseases, which can cause disabilities in humans, limit their productivity in society, and negatively affect their quality of life [1–5].

In all societies, blindness has profound human and socioeconomic consequences. The costs of loss of productivity, rehabilitation, and education for the blind constitute a significant economic burden for the individual, the family, and society [6].

Thus, it is interesting to know that total or partial opacification of the lens is the main cause of bilateral blindness and severe visual impairment represents about 48% of cases of visual impairment in the world and is known to have a multifactorial cause. In addition, it incapacitates the individual and increases their dependence and early retirement from life [7].

2. Classification

According to the WHO, visual function is subdivided into four levels: normal vision, moderate visual impairment, severe visual impairment, and blindness. Visual disability includes moderate and severe visual impairment and blindness [8, 9], see **Table 1**.

Category	Visual acuity
Normal vision	20/20–20/60
Moderate visual impairment	20/60–20/200
Severe visual disability	20/200–20/400
Blindness	≥20/400
	Count the fingers at 1, 2, 3 m
	HM
	PL
	DNPL

Symbology: Hand movement (HM), perceive light (PL), do not perceive light (DNPL), meter (m).

Table 1.
Classification of visual function according to the WHO.

The International Classification of Diseases (WHO ICD-10) contains the following definitions:

1. Blindness: visual acuity (AV) less than 20/400 in the best eye with the available correction (AVCD), with the best possible correction AVMC or with pinhole hole (AVAE)

2. Severe visual impairment (DVG): AV 20/200–20/400 in the best eye with the AVCD, AVMC, or AVAE

3. Moderate visual impairment (MVD): AV 20/60–20/200 in the best eye with AVCD, AVMC, or AVAE [7, 10, 11]

4. Low vision: alteration of visual function, even after treatment and/or standard correction of refraction and an AV less than 20/60 to perception of light but useful for planning or executing a task [7, 8, 10, 11]

3. Epidemiology

According to the WHO data, it is estimated that, worldwide, approximately 1300 million people live with some form of visual impairment. More than 314 million have a severe visual impairment. Of these, 37 million are blind and 124 million suffer from low vision. Eighty percent of all these cases are considered avoidable [12, 13].

According to WHO estimates, of the more than 26 million people with visual disorders in the Region of the Americas in 2010, more than 3 million were blind, and most of them were 50 years of age or older [12].

Most of the national and local surveys were published and published in Latin America, and refractive errors were not corrected in the main cause of visual impairment, both severe (19.7%) and moderate (58.6%) [14–16].

Between 1990 and 2010, the prevalences normalized according to the age of blindness, and moderate and severe visual impairment decreased in Latin America and the Caribbean [17].

The WHO estimated the prevalence of blindness in 2002 in people over 50 years by subregions [18], see **Table 2**. In Latin America, the prevalence of blindness in people over 50 responds between 1% in urban areas with good socioeconomic

WHO subregion	Country	Prevalence of blindness in people aged 50+ (%)
Amr-A	Canada, Cuba, USA	0.4
Amr-B	Argentina, Bahamas, Belize, Brazil, Chile, Colombia, Costa Rica, Dominica, Dominican Republic, El Salvador, Grenada, Guyana, Honduras, Jamaica, Mexico, Panama, Paraguay, Suriname, Uruguay, Venezuela	1.3
Amr-C	Bolivia, Ecuador, Guatemala, Haiti, Nicaragua, Peru	2.6

Source: Silva [18].

Table 2.
Estimates of the prevalence of blindness in 2002 in people over 50 years of age by subregion of the WHO.

Country	Uncorrected refractive error (%)	Uncorrected cataract (%)	Non-trachomatous corneal opacity (%)	Glaucoma (%)	Diabetic retinopathy (%)	Age-related macular degeneration (%)
Argentina	8.0	44.0	0.0	8.0	16.0	4.0
El Salvador	4.0	68.7	7.1	5.1	5.1	4.0
Honduras	3.0	59.2	2.6	21.1	0.0	3.9
Panamá	0.1	66.4	2.2	10.2	1.5	5.1
Paraguay	3.1	43.8	9.4	15.6	6.3	9.4
Peru	1.5	58.0	5.3	13.7	0.8	11.5
Uruguay	2.9	48.6	0.0	14.3	5.7	8.6

Source: Silva [23].

Table 3.
Main reported causes of blindness adults over 50 years, Latin America, 2011–2013.

development and more than 4% in rural and marginal areas [19]. In Central America, the prevalence of blindness is 2.1% (95% CI: 1.7–2.7) [17], and in countries such as Panama, it is 3.0% (95% CI: 2.3–3.6) [20], Costa Rica 1.7% (2.1%, IC95%: 1.7–2.7) [21], and Honduras 1.9% (95% CI: 1.4–2.4%) [22].

In Latin America, cataract without correction represents by far the main cause of blindness in adults over 50 years, followed by glaucoma, diabetic retinopathy (DR), age-related macular degeneration, and uncorrected refractive errors [23], see **Table 3**.

4. Etiology

The causes from one country to another. The visual impairment attributable to cataract is greater in low- and middle-income countries than in high-income countries. In high-income countries, diseases such as diabetic retinopathy, glaucoma, and macular degeneration are related to the most frequent age [24].

Johns Hopkins University has found that the main cause of blindness in white people is macular degeneration associated with age, while in the black population, it is due to glaucoma or cataract. In addition, in the elderly, blindness is three times more frequent in blacks than in whites [25].

Causes	Definition
Cataract	It is the opacity of the lens, which is understood as the passage of light to the retina, causes a slow and progressive loss of vision, and can appear at any stage of life, from birth to older age than being human [27–30]
Glaucoma	It is an optic neuropathy that presents with a characteristic structural damage, associated with the progressive death of retinal ganglion cells, loss of nerve fibers, and loss of pathognomonic visual field [31–34]
Uncorrected refraction	In myopia, the point of focus is in front of the retina, because the cornea has too much curvature or the axial length of the eye is excessive In hyperopia, the focus point is behind the retina because the cornea has too flat a curvature or the axial length is too short Astigmatism, a non-spherical (variable) curvature of the cornea or lens, causes light rays of different orientations (e.g., vertical, oblique, horizontal) to focus on different points [35] Presbyopia is a clinical loss of the amplitude of accommodation or, in other words, the loss of the ability to change the shape of the lens to focus on nearby objects [35, 36]

Table 4.
The most common causes of visual disability and blindness.

The main causes of blindness in order of frequency are cataract (39%), uncorrected refractive errors (18%), glaucoma (10%), macular degeneration related to age (7%), corneal opacities (4%), diabetic retinopathy (4%), trachoma (3%), childhood eye diseases (3%), and onchocerciasis (0.7%). Cataract is the leading cause of easily curable blindness [7, 26].

For this reason, a description of the main causes is made, see **Table 4**.

5. Risk factors

The different etiologies are known to have multifactorial causes; in cataract modifiable risk factors are identified as exposure to ultraviolet rays, mainly UV-B, deficiency in the diet of antioxidants and proteins, smoking, diabetes mellitus, the use of corticosteroids, and severe dehydration. And non-modifiable risk factors are genetic, with a probability three times higher in relatives of people with the disease [37–41].

In glaucoma it is said that age increases the probability of suffering ocular hypertension. A glaucoma can evolve of various etiologies. The prevalence increases from 4 to 10 times in people older than 60 years [42]. Other risk factors are myopia, inheritance, African-American race, exfoliation, and pigmentary dispersion [43].

Refractive errors are associated with racial factors, the myopia and astigmatism are more prevalent in the Chinese population and hyperopia is the most common in the Hispanic population [44].

Regarding diabetic retinopathy (DR), it corresponds to one of the microvascular complications of diabetes mellitus.

The risk factors are the time of evolution of DM and poor glycemic control, glycosylated hemoglobin (HbA1c) level greater than 6.9% [45], associated arterial hypertension [46, 47], juvenile type 2 DM of early onset [48], and genetic susceptibility (the haptoglobin genotype 1-1) [49].

In **Figure 1**, the relationship between glycemic control and the duration of diabetes with diabetic retinopathy is shown as a function of the time of follow-up, with different curves for the different HbA1C values [50].

Between 80 and 95% corresponds to simple or nonproliferative DR and the remaining 5–10% to proliferative DR [51].

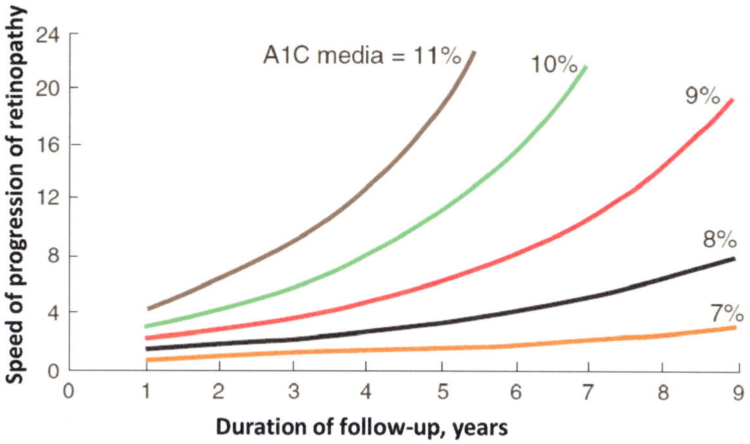

Figure 1.
The relationship between glycemic control and duration of diabetes with diabetic retinopathy. Source: Longo et al. [50].

6. Differential diagnosis

Basic knowledge of ocular symptoms is required to perform an adequate ophthalmological evaluation. It is always necessary to completely define the characteristics of the symptoms and discomforts.

The ocular symptoms can be classified in the fundamental categories: abnormalities of the eyes, anomalies of the ocular aspect and abnormalities of the sensations, pains, and ocular discomforts.

Therefore, it can be useful to make one order and ask the following questions:

1. Has the disorder **started** gradually, quickly, or asymptomatically? For example, was blurred vision in one eye discovered until the other eye was inadvertently covered?

2. Was the **duration** of the problem brief, or did the symptom persist until the current consultation? If the symptom has been intermittent, how has been its frequency?

3. Is the **location** of the disorder focal or diffuse, and is it a unilateral or bilateral condition? Finally, does the patient rate the degree of the disorder as mild, moderate, or severe?

In **Table 5**, some of the main characteristics of the most common pathologies associated with preventable blindness are observed.

6.1 Physical exam

Of all the organs of the body, the eye is the most accessible to direct examination. The visual function can be evaluated by means of simple subjective tests. The same can be taken care of from an adequate primary care service.

The clinic plays a decisive role in the initial evaluation of any patient, so the correct approach orderly and systematic is essential in the sequence of subsequent processes for the consolidation of a presumptive diagnosis and complementary tests and to achieve an accurate diagnosis and therapeutic approach suitable.

Clinic	Cataract [52]	Uncorrected refraction [53]	Glaucoma [54, 55]	
			Primary open-angle glaucoma	**Closed-angle glaucoma**
			60–70%	10%
Evolution	Chronicle		Chronicle Asymptomatic until very advanced phases Discovery is usually casual	Acute Preceded intermittent attacks, or else it occurs suddenly It represents a true ophthalmological emergency
Visual acuity	Decreases progressively	• Myopia, difficulty to see clearly distant objects • Long-range difficulty to clearly see nearby objects • Astigmatism or distorted vision • Presbyopia, difficulty reading or focusing well in the distance	Losses of the visual field: central vision is the last to be affected, peripheral vision is lost first	Decreases
Blurry vision	Present	Present		
Pain			There may be headaches and eye pain	Intense pain in the distribution zone of the V cranial nerve
Diplopia	Present			
Symmetry of affectation			Bilateral and asymmetric	Unilateral but both eyes are susceptible to affectation in different evolutionary moments
Association	With presbyopia and myopia			With vegetative symptoms (profuse sweating, nausea, vomiting, tachycardia, etc.)

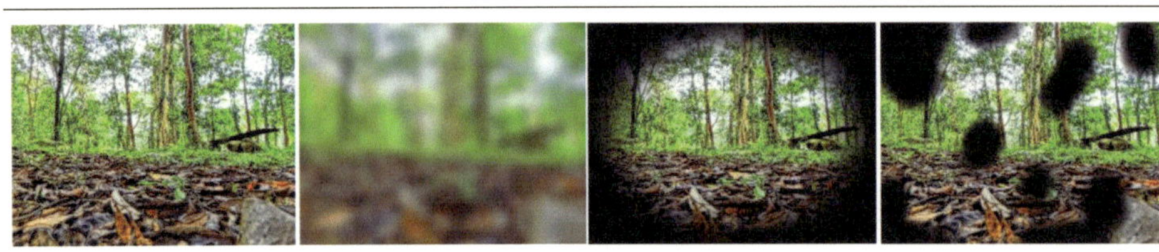

Table 5.
Clinic of the main causes of visual disability and blindness.

Therefore, an adequate anamnesis that includes general, sociodemographic data, personal and family pathological history, and ocular and non-ocular as well as traumatic surgical history is imperative and invariably its symptomatology.

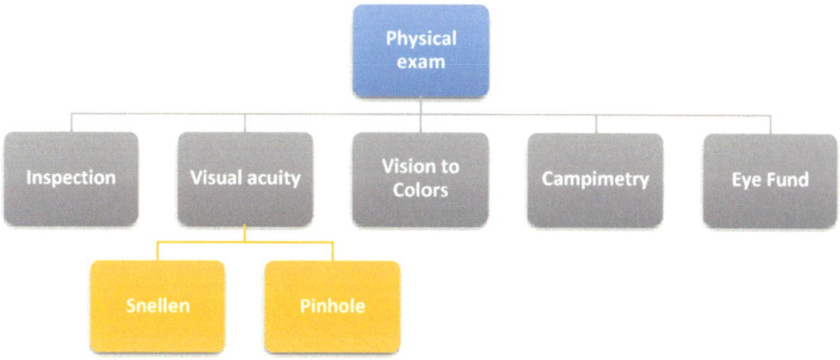

Figure 2.
Basic ophthalmologic exploration.

Physical examination	
Cataract [56]	Opacification of the lens Pupillary reflexes may be slowed down, but they do not disappear
Uncorrected refraction [52]	Improvement of the AV with the pinhole hole test
Glaucoma [54, 55]	Closed-angle glaucoma • Conjunctival and ciliary injection • Corneal edema with loss of transparency of the cornea • Difficult to visualize the details of the iris compared to the contralateral eye • Oval ovarian suture in a reactive mean mydriasis • The eye is hard (stony) to pressure
Diabetic retinopathy [57]	Vascular microaneurysms, hemorrhage, cotton-wool exudates, vein caliber alterations, neovascularizations

Table 6.
Findings of the physical examination in the main causes of visual disability and blindness.

The external anatomy of the eye is visible and can be examined with the naked eye or with simple instruments.

The eye is the only part of the body where you have direct vision to blood vessels and tissues of the central nervous system (retina and optic nerve). Thanks to this it is possible to identify, by ocular examination, important systemic effects of infectious, autoimmune, neoplastic, and vascular diseases.

And so, a basic physical examination aimed at the search of suspected abnormalities that merit its timely reference to a higher level of specialty is essential in the primary care physician, see **Figure 2**.

And it is in this sense that it can describe certain characteristic findings of these pathologies, the same ones that can guide our mental scheme to achieve a presumptive diagnosis; some of them are described in **Table 6**.

7. Prevention

The Latin America and the Caribbean region are considered one of the most inequitable in the world in terms of the distribution of goods and services, social determinants, and health.

Using a standard methodology for international use [58], it has been possible to determine the prevalence of blindness and visual impairment, coverage, and the quality of cataract services and barriers to access them in several countries [56].

The Vision 2020 program in Latin America, with the participation of PAHO/WHO, the Christian Blind Mission, and the International Agency for the Prevention of Blindness, has proposed to document the problem of blindness and visual impairment in people over 50 years of age and designed a statistical instrument called "rapid assessment of avoidable blindness" (ERCE). To date, ERCE activities have been conducted to determine the prevalence of blindness [16, 49, 50–63].

And it is through this instrument that in nine countries of Latin America, the following barriers have been determined for cataract surgery: lack of knowledge about the existence of a treatment, it is thought to be the destination, there is no availability of surgery services or very distant, fear of the operation or loss of vision, cannot pay for the operation, indication of waiting until it "matures" (possible waiting list), no one can accompany to the ophthalmological care, and other diseases and contraindications for surgery [64–66].

All are surmountable through information and education campaigns.

8. Conclusions

To control blindness and visual impairment, it is essential to implement plans to (a) detect cases of low vision and operate cataract cases, (b) detect and give optical correction to cases with refractive errors and presbyopia, and (c) integrate eye care in primary health care. These three interventions could solve around 67% of cases of blindness and could help detect people with glaucoma, in order to treat them in early stages.

Eighty percent of all these cases are considered avoidable. Therefore, the exhaustive evaluation in the patient with determining risks plays a key role, together with the fact that the visual function can be evaluated by means of simple subjective tests and be attended to by an adequate primary care service.

The difficulties in the supply of surgeries vary according to the country, being very available for most of the population in developed countries and becoming the most performed surgery in the elderly. In developing countries, the situation varies according to the regions or countries.

Visual disability and blindness correspond to one of the microvascular complications of diabetes mellitus, where the relationship that keeps the glycemic control in function of the time of presenting the disease is widely demonstrated. Between 80 and 95% corresponds to nonproliferative DR and the remaining 5–10% to proliferative DR. Here is the need for a holistic approach to the patient aimed at prevention and proper medical management.

Author details

Mercedes Libeth Ramos Amador and Javier Eduardo Escober Torres*
Doctor of Medicine and Surgery National Autonomous University of Honduras, Tegucigalpa, Honduras

*Address all correspondence to: jetorres.9307@gmail.com

References

[1] Rodríguez Masó S, Rojas Rondón I, Vázquez Adán Y, Venereo Rodríguez A, Baute Puerto B, Landrove Y. Caracterización clinico-epidemiológica de la baja visión en el adulto mayor y su rehabilitación visual. Revista Cubana de Oftalmología. 2014;**27**(3):416-426

[2] López-Alemany A, Uson E. Low vision and contact lenses. Revista Española de Contactología. 2007;**14**(14):8. ISSN: 1989-7111. Available from: http://www.oftalmo.com/sec/07-tomo-1/03.htm

[3] Bayarre H, Pérez Piñero J, Menéndez Jiménez J. Las transiciones demográficas, epidemiológicas y la calidad de vida objetiva en la tercera edad. GEROINFO. 2006;**1**:1-34. Available from: http://www.sld.cu/galerias/pdf/sitios/gericuba/las_transiciones_demograficaepidemiologica_y_la_calidad_de_vida_objetiva_en_la_tercera_edad.pdf

[4] Salomao SR, Cinoto RW, Berezovsky A, Araujo-Filho A, Mitsuhiro MR, Mendieta L, et al. Prevalence and causes of vision impairment and blindness in older adults in Brazil: The Sao Paulo eye study. Ophthalmic Epidemiology. 2008;**15**(3):167-175

[5] Moreno Domínguez JC, De la Portilla Castro MM, Correa Rojas O, Iviricu Tielves R, Sanabria NJ. Afecciones visuales y su tratamiento en la población de Pinar del Río, Misión Milagro de 2006-2010. Revista Cubana de Oftalmología. 2012;**25**(2):264-277

[6] Rojas H et al. Catarata, una causa prevenible de ceguera. Revista Médica Hondureña. 2014;**82**(4):160-163

[7] World Health Organization. Global Initiative for the Elimination of Avoidable Blindness: Action Plan 2006-2011. Geneva: WHO; 2007

[8] OMS. Ceguera y Discapacidad Visual Organización Mundial de la Salud. Nota Descriptiva No. 282. 2018. Available from: https://www.who.int/es/newsroom/ fact-sheets/detail/blindnessand-visual-impairment

[9] OMS. Change the Definition of Blindness. Definitions of Blindness and Visual Impairment. Ginebra: Organización Mundial de la Salud; 2012

[10] World Health Organization. Change the Definition of Blindness [En Internet]. 2014. Disponible en: http://www.who.int/blindness/Change%20the%20Definition%20of%20Blindness.pdf [Consultado el 17 de abril del 2019]

[11] Guisasola L et al. Informe de la Salud Visual en Suramérica. Cátedra Unesco de Salud Visual y Desarrollo. 2008. Available from: https://unescovision.upc.edu/es/materiales/materiales-de-lacatedra/investigacion/savim/informe-de-la-salud-visual-en-sudamerica-2008

[12] World Health Organization. Global Data on Visual Impairment 2010. Geneva: WHO; 2012. WHO/NMH/PBD/12.01. Disponible en: http://www.who.int/blindness/GLOBALDATAFINALforweb.pdf

[13] Eckert K. Visión 2020 América Latina. Plan Estratégico [Internet]. Ginebra: OMS; 2012. Available from: http://www.v2020la.org/images/Plan_Estrategico_2012.pdf [Cited: April 05, 2019]

[14] Lewallen S, Perez-Straziota C, Lansingh V, Limburg H, Silva JC. Variation in cataract surgery needs in Latin America. Archives of Ophthalmology. 2012;**130**(12):1575-1578. DOI: 10.1001/archophthalmol.2012.2147

[15] Kuper H, Polack S, Limburg H. Rapid assessment of avoidable blindness. Community Eye Health. 2006;**19**(60):68-69

[16] Pongo Águila L, Carrión R, Luna W, Silva JC, Limburg H. Cataract blindness in people 50 years old or older in a semirural area of Northern Peru. The Revista Panamericana de Salud Pública. 2005;**17**(5-6):387-393

[17] Leasher JL, Lansingh V, Flaxman SM, Jonas JB, Keeffe J, Naidoo K, et al. Prevalence and causes of vision loss in Latin America and the Caribbean: 1990-2010. The British Journal of Ophthalmology. 2014;**98**(5):619-628

[18] Silva JC. Review of recent surveys on blindness and visual impairment in Latin America. British Journal of Ophthalmology. 2008;**92**(3):315-319

[19] Consejo Directivo OPS. Plan de Acción para la Prevención de la de la Ceguera y de las Deficiencias Visuales. 154.a Sesión del Comité Ejecutivo. Washington: OPS; 2014. 20p

[20] López M, Brea I, Yee R, Yi R, Carles V, Broce A, et al. Encuesta de ceguera y deficiencia visual evitable en Panamá. Revista Panamericana de Salud Pública. 2014;**36**(6):355-360

[21] Acevedo R, Carranza E, Cortés R, Rodríguez G. Estimación de la prevalencia de enfermedades asociadas a ceguera prevenible y discapacidad visual en Costa Rica para el año 2015 [Tesis] [Internet]. Costa Rica: Médico Especialista en Oftalmología, Universidad de Costa Rica. Sistema de Estudios de Posgrado; 2016. Disponible en: http://repositorio.sibdi.ucr.ac.cr:8080/jspui/handle/123456789/5321 [Citado 2019 Jun 19]

[22] Alvarado D, Rivera B, Lagos L, Ochoa M, Starkman I, Castillo M, et al. Encuesta nacional de ceguera y deficiencia visual evitables en Honduras. Revista Panamericana de Salud Pública. 2014;**36**(5):300-305

[23] Silva JC. Una evaluación comparativa de la ceguera y la deficiencia visual evitables en siete países latinoamericanos, prevalencia cobertura y desigualdades. Revista Panamericana de Salud Pública. 2015;**37**(1):21-28

[24] OMS. Ceguera y Discapacidad Visual [Internet]. 2018. Disponible en: www.who.int/es/news-room/fact-sheets/detail/blindness-and-visual-impairment [Citado 2019 abril 06]

[25] Highlights of Ophthalmology International. Encuentran diferencias raciales relacionadas con la ceguera. Revista Archives of Ophthalmology. 2006;**20**(2). ISSN 0864-2176

[26] World Health Organization. Action Plan for the Prevention of Avoidable Blindness and Visual Impairment 2009-2013. Geneva: WHO; 2010

[27] Merino G. Escuela de Medicina UDA Oftalmología. Curso de Oftalmología 5to año. Catarata [Serie en Internet]. 2002. Disponible en: http://www.escuela.med.puc.cl [Citado 12 de mayo de 2007]

[28] Alemañy Martorell J. Oftalmología. La Habana: Editorial Ciencias Médicas; 2005. pp. 179-186

[29] American Academy of Ophthalmology. Cataract in the Adult Eye. Preferred Practice Patterns. USA: AAO Anterior Segment Panel; 2001

[30] Kanski JJ, Menon J. Oftalmología Clínica. 5th ed. España: Editorial Elsevier España; 2005. p. 165-194, 448-465, 698-700

[31] Taylor HR, Keeffe JE. World blindness: A 21st century perspective. British Journal of Ophthalmology. 2001;**85**:261-266

[32] Coleman AL. Glaucoma. Lancet. 1999;**354**:1803-1819. DOI: 10.1016/S0140-6736(99)04240-3

[33] Quigley H. How common is glaucoma worldwide? International Glaucoma Review. 2002;**3**(3):11-12

[34] Mardin CY, Junemman AGM. The diagnostic value of imaging in early glaucoma. Current Opinion in Ophthalmology. 2001;**12**:100-104

[35] Dhaliwal DK. Generalidades de los Defectos de la Refracción. Manual MSD [Internet]. 2017. Disponible en: https://www.msdmanuals.com/es/professional/trastornos-oftálmicos/defectos-de-la-refracción/generalidades-de-los-defectos-de-la-refracción [Citado 2019 Abril 15]

[36] Glasser A, Campbell MCW. Presbyopia and the optical changes in the human crystalline lens with age. Vision Research. 1998;**38**(2):209-229

[37] Leite Arieta CE, Duerksen R, Lansingh V. Manual de Ceguera Por Catarata en América Latina. Bogotá: Imagen & Diseño producciones Ltda; 2011

[38] Lindblad BE, Håkansson N, Wolk A. Smoking cessation and the risk of cataract: A prospective cohort study of cataract extraction among men. JAMA Ophthalmology. 2014;**132**(3):253-257

[39] Wu R, Wang JJ, Mitchell P, Lamoureux EL, Zheng Y, Rochtchina E, et al. Smoking, socioeconomic factors, and age-related cataract: The Singapore Malay eye study. Archives of Ophthalmology. 2010;**128**(8):1029-1035

[40] Rautiainen S, Lindblad BE, Morgenstern R, Wolk A. Total antioxidant capacity of the diet and risk of age-related cataract: A population-based prospective cohort of women. JAMA Ophthalmology. 2014;**132**(3):247-252

[41] Robin AL, Thulasiraj RD. Cataract blindness. Archives of Ophthalmology. 2012;**130**(11):1452-1455

[42] Courtright P. Género y salud ocular. Salud Ocular Comunitaria. 2010;**4**(8):10-12. ISSN 1993-7229

[43] Van Veldhuisen PC. et al, The advanced Glaucoma Intervention Study (AGIS): The relationship between control of intraocular pressure and visual field deterioration. American Journal of Ophthalmology. 2000;**130**:429-440

[44] Pan CW, Klein BE, Cotch MF, et al. Racial variations in the prevalence of refractive errors in the United States: The multi-ethnic study of atherosclerosis. American Journal of Ophthalmology. 2013;**155**:1129-1138. DOI: 10.1016/j.ajo.2013.01.009

[45] Saum SL, Thomas E, Lewis AM, Croft PR. The effect of diabetic control on the incidence of, and changes in, retinopathy in type 2 non-insulin dependent diabetic patients. The British Journal of General Practice. 2002;**52**(476):214-216

[46] Herold P, Craig ME, Hing S, Donaghue K. Role of blood pressure in development of early retinopathy in adolescents with type 1 diabetes: Prospective cohort study. BMJ. 2008;**337**:a918

[47] Wong TY, Mitchell P. The eye in hypertension. Lancet. 2007;**369**(9559):425-435

[48] Wong J, Molyneaux L, Constantino M, Twigg SM, Yue DK. Timing is everything: Age of onset influences long-term retinopathy risk in type 2 diabetes, independent of traditional risk factors. Diabetes Care. 2008;**31**(10):1985-1990

[49] Nakhoul FM, Marsh S, Hochberg I, Leibu R, Miller BP, Levy AP.

Haptoglobin genotype as a risk factor for diabetic retinopathy. Journal of the American Medical Association. 2000;**284**(10):1244-1245

[50] Longo DL, Fauci AS, Kasper DL, Hauser SL, Jameson JL, Loscalzo J, editors. Harrison Principios de Medicina Interna. 18th ed. Vol. 2. México: McGraw-Hill; 2012. p. 2981

[51] Rodriguez J, Sanchez R, Munoz B, West SK, Broman A, Snyder RW, et al. Causes of blindness and visual impairment in a population-based sample of U.S. Hispanics. Ophthalmology. 2002;**109**(4):737-743

[52] Garbín Fuentes I, Pérez Chica G. Patología del Cristalino. Cataratas. Disponible en: http://www.sepeap.org/archivos/libros/OFTALMOLOGIA/Ar_1844APR8.pdf [Fecha de acceso. 15 de mayo del 2019]

[53] Vicente T, Ramirez M, de la Torre I, Garcia L, Lopez A, Terradillos M, et al. Prevalencia de defectos visuales en trabajadores españoles. Repercusión de Variables Sociodemográficas y Laborales. 2016;**90**(2):49-100. Disponible en: https://www.elsevier.es/es-revista-revista-mexicana-oftalmologia-321-articulo-prevalencia-defectos-visuales-trabajadores-espanoles--S0187451915000931

[54] Piñeiro RT, Lora M, Andres MI. Glaucoma. Offarm. 2005;**22**:88-96

[55] González del Valle F. Sección I: Oftalmología. In: Diagnóstico y Tratamiento Médico. Oftalmología General. Vaughan & Asbury. Mexico: McGraw-Hill; 2011. pp. 230-245. Chapter 11. ISBN: 978-0-07-163420-5

[56] Mura J. Cirugía actual de la catarata. Departamento de Oftalmología, Clínica Las Condes. 2010;**21**(6):864-1005. Disponible en: https://www.elsevier.es/es-revista-revista-medica-clinica-las-condes-202-articulo-cirugia-actual-catarata-S0716864010706155

[57] Mohamed Q, Gillies MC, Wong TY. Management of diabetic retinopathy: A systematic review. Journal of the American Medical Association. 2007;**298**(8):902-916

[58] Pan American Health Organization. Health in the Americas, 2012 ed. Regional Outlook and Country Profiles. Washington: PAHO; 2012

[59] Kuper H, Polack S, Limburg H. Rapid assessment of avoidable blindness. Community Eye Health. 2006;**19**:68-69

[60] Limburg H, Meester W, Hannah K, Polack S. ERCE 5 Manual de Evaluación Rápida de la Ceguera Evitable. Reino Unido: Centro Internacional de Salud Ocular; 2012

[61] Limburg H, Barria von-Bischhoffshausen F, Gomez P, Silva JC, Foster A. Review of recent surveys on blindness and visual impairment in Latin America. The British Journal of Ophthalmology. 2008;**92**(3):315-319

[62] Nano ME, Nano HD, Mugica JM, Silva JC, Montaña G, Limburg H. Rapid assessment of visual impairment due to cataract and cataract surgical services in urban Argentina. Ophthalmic Epidemiology. 2006;**13**(3):191-197

[63] Beltranena F, Casasola K, Silva JC, Limburg H. Cataract blindness in 4 regions of Guatemala: Results of a population-based survey. Ophthalmology. 2007;**114**(8):1558-1563

[64] Limburg H, Silva JC, Foster A. Cataract in Latin America: Findings from nine recent surveys. The Revista Panamericana de Salud Pública. 2009;**25**(5):449-455

[65] Suárez Escudero JC. Discapacidad visual y ceguera en el adulto: Revisión de tema. Medicina UPB. 2011;**30**(2):170-180

[66] Burga HG, Hinds CN, Lansingh VC, Samudio M, Lewallen S, Courtright P, et al. Is the cost the primary barrier for cataract surgery in Paraguay? Arquivos Brasileiros de Oftalmologia. 2014;77(3):164-167

Section 2

Public Health

Chapter 6

Role of Primary Health Care System in Response to a Major Incident: Challenges and Actions

Abdulnasir Falah Huaidi Al-Jazairi

Abstract

There is obvious increase in world population and in term of number of major incidents (MI) all over the world, there is a need for faster and wider responses. To achieve this aim and keep losses to the minimum, we need to optimize our methods and protocols of the response to decrease the losses, pain, and suffering of people and losses of infrastructures, belongings, and the country's future. Primary health care (PHC) system, which is present in all residency gatherings in cities and towns, provides suitable potential for this improvement. This role has been formulated in 1978 in Alma-Ata meeting, which changes the scope of service of primary health care system to take responsibility of the community in addition to patients' care. The involvement of the primary health care in response to major incidents shows good results, and there is a need to strengthen the major incidents' response plan in the primary health care to provide better response and help to all populations especially the vulnerable ones.

Keywords: primary health care, major incidents, vulnerable population, planning, response, recovery

1. Introduction

There is a noticeable increase in major incidents (MI) of different types affecting the world in the last three decades with increased human and financial losses. There are different types of incidents: natural, man-made, and infectious epidemics. For optimum response to those incidents, there should be multidisciplinary coordinated teams' response [1].

Shortly after I started writing this chapter, the COVID-19 epidemic in China expanded to be a pandemic, affecting too many countries and hundreds of thousands of people and killing more than 50,000 all over the world. This has a clear effect on my chapter to concentrate on this type of major incidents.

Primary health care (PHC) system scope of service was concentrated on disease consultations and prescription of medication. This scope had been changed in 1978 by the Declaration of Alma-Ata, which considered health care as fundamental human right. Section V in the declaration stated clearly that the primary health care system is the key to achieve the targets of the declaration. This declaration leads to the change of the scope of work of the PHC from giving advice about patients' symptoms to the comprehensive health care of the community [2]. This aim of comprehensive health care of the PHC was reviewed in WHO report in 2008 [3], which centered on taking the PHC service from hospitals and specialized centers to be nearby people in general walk-in clinics that are easily reached by community. This proved to have many benefits in:

- Relief suffering
- Prevention of illness and death
- Improved health equity

The PHC system, with its distribution in all areas to be near to large population, can play an important role in response to any MI affecting its catchment area. The PHC staff have better knowledge in their area population and the special needs categories. Those abilities enable the PHC system to play a crucial role in response to major incidents in all their stages.

2. Definitions

2.1 Primary health care system

PHC is a whole-of-society approach to health that aims to ensure the highest possible level of health and well-being and their equitable distribution by focusing on people's needs and preferences (as individuals, families, and communities) as early as possible along the continuum from health promotion and disease prevention to treatment, rehabilitation, and palliative care and as close as feasible to people's everyday environment [4].

2.2 Comprehensive health care

"The practice of continuing comprehensive care is the concurrent prevention and management of multiple physical and emotional health problems of a patient over a period of time in relationship to family, life events and environment" [5].

2.3 Major incident

In health care system, "A major incident can be defined as any incident where the location, number, severity or type of live casualties requires extraordinary resources" [6].

2.4 Vulnerable populations

Vulnerable populations include patients who are racial or ethnic minorities, children, elderly, socioeconomically disadvantaged, underinsured, or those with certain medical conditions. Members of **vulnerable populations** often have health conditions that are exacerbated by unnecessarily inadequate health care [7].

3. Factors that make PHC suitable to play an essential role in response to MI

- **Work concept**: Changing to comprehensive health care of the community makes the PHC responsible to prepare people to a disaster if there is time to and help them during its occurrence and in the post-incident stage.

- **Community based**: The responsibility is for the welfare of the whole community and not for medical advice when asked only.
- **Easy accessibility**: The presence of PHC centers in close proximity to people makes them reachable with little efforts. During a major incident, there are many things people are busy with, or some have lost helpers; the presence of a nearby health care facility will decrease patients and people suffering in attending and getting the proper health advice they need.
- **Dealing with all types of diseases**: The PHC centers are run by family medicine physicians (FP) or general practitioners (GP), and they are trained to deal with all types of diseases and possess the ability to deal with all patients or persons asking different types of consultations in many specialties.
- **Filtering ability**: The doctors in primary care are trained to deal with patients in all specialties. This practice gives them the ability to work in the early step of sorting cases. PHC can deal with simple cases that constitute 50 to 60% of cases and keep hospitals and specialized centers for more severe cases.
- **Decrease cost**: FP/GP use less tools and request less investigations for their work, and this cuts the cost the patient should pay for care. This is exaggerated during major incident circumstances, which enable the health system to deal with larger number of patients in the same cost if the patients have been managed by hospitals only.

Stages of major incidents: Most of the researchers divide the major incidents into four stages:

A. Mitigation and prevention

B. Preparedness

C. Response

D. Recovery

Although this has many positive implications, Quarantelli in 1980 [8] put major incident phases depending on the time factor. He put three phases as follows:

I. Pre-impact phase

II. Trans-impact phase

III. Post-impact phase

In the coming sections, I will discuss the role of the PHC system according to the phase and regarding the staff, space, stuff, and communication roles. The discussion will be divided into two parts as follows:

A. **Effect of major incident on primary health care.** This will be under the title "Challenges."

B. **Actions by the primary health care in response.** This will be under the title "Actions."

4. Pre-impact phase

PHC system is the nearest health facility to most people and is easily accessible; therefore, it is, mostly, the first place that the patients will attend to get information and advice for their conditions and worries about any new threat or risk.

4.1 Challenges

The challenges will affect PHC staff and PHC facility. The challenges will depend on the risks more suspected in the geographical area in which the health facility is present.

4.1.1 PHC staff

a. The PHC staff are holding double personality during major incidents; from one side they are part of families and they have responsibilities for them, and on the other side, they have commitment to work to help people and other community services.

b. The staff will be under pressure to have answers to the new threat and its relations to the different diseases and medications.

c. Dealing with major incidents is not part of day-to-day activity of the health sector; therefore, there is lack of knowledge of the major incident response plan (MIRP) to the facility and their specific roles. All staff in the PHC in all levels whether clinical or nonclinical should have specific training on the MIRP and their specific role in it, so everybody will speak the same language during the response and can harmonize work better.

d. Psychiatric aspect of the major incident will affect both PHC staff and people visiting the health facility. Staff should have basic training to deal with those difficult situations.

4.1.2 PHC facility

a. There will be an increase in visits to PHC from people for different consultations, which will lead to overcrowding in the PHC.

b. More medications and stuff are requested by patients to have stocks during the expected incidents. This will impose pressure on the stocks of the medications and consumable stuffs.

c. How to change the layout of the facility to accommodate more visitors if needed? This is depending on the blue print of the facility and whether it is manageable or not.

d. Is the facility in danger of the incident or not? This is more applicable in the natural disasters like earthquake, tornados, and hurricanes. What to do if it is affected and cannot provide service?

e. The infrastructures like electricity, water, or network may be affected by the incident. What are the substitutes or mitigation solutions for this breakdown?

4.2 Actions

The period before expected incidents is a suitable situation to do improvements in planning, training for staff, and stockpiling stuff. PHC administrators need to achieve the following aims:

a. Orient the local and national health system on the PHC active involvement in protecting community, and strengthen the skills of risk management in the PHC directors.

b. Concentrate on efforts to support communities, individuals, and health workers to better respond to major incidents. This is done by providing enough information about the disease and protective measures, vaccinations, and actions to do if any family member or oneself is affected.

c. Financial investment in the infrastructures of the PHC regarding water, electricity, information, communications, and supply network.

The abovementioned aims will be accomplished through the following:

4.3 Planning

PHC should work in close collaboration with local health authority and other emergency services in developing response plans.

They should look to the following issues:

1. Define hazards and risk factors to the area, in collaboration with other emergency services. This will help in predicting expected incidents and their effects on the health of the community they are serving. Also, it will help in preparing the type of medications and consumables.

2. Make lists with addresses of the vulnerable population and those using regular medications in their area. This will allow the health and other authorities to prepare shelter, medications, and other care plans during MI.

3. The effect of the expected MI on different diseases should be prepared with the help of the specialized sections in local, state, or federal (or ministerial) health authorities. Information should be relayed to the concerned patients along with best mitigation actions.

4. Setting agreements with ambulance services to transfer patients (who need hospital transfer) received in PHC during MI.

5. Information regarding any MI expected, its nature, the expected size, and the need to activate the MI response plan. That critical information should be verified, i.e., the source of information should be trusted and accurate.

6. Allocate area to be an alternative place, and make pre-arrangement for rapid conversion into PHC facility if the original building became unsuitable for work.

4.4 Training staff

Staff should have training on several aspects of MI response including the needed information to help the community and individuals.

This includes the following:

1. Training the staff on the MI response plan set for the area. The response plan should be flexible to meet the different types and effects of different incidents. The plan should rhyme with the local and state health response plan.

2. Training the staff on communication with people including agitated and aggressive people. Communication training should include breaking bad news. They may have to visit families and inform them about their relatives, good or bad news.

3. Training on working in austere conditions in case there is damage to the infrastructure of the PHC facility and a need to work in small or large teams depending on the incident circumstances and decision of the local authority or state's incident response leaders.

4. Training on more than one method of communication including radio communication protocols. Radio communication will be used if other methods are lost by the effect of the incident.

4.5 Prepare for infrastructure failure

a. Electricity failure is one of the major failures during MI. It has serious negative effects on patients' care. Electricity generator working on petrol should be prepared and maintained regularly to be ready anytime electricity cut occurs.

b. Water loss. Large water reservoir should be ready, and the water should be replaced on a daily basis. In addition, drinking water bottles should be part of stockpiling in preparation to a major incident. Potable drinking water in addition to clean water suitable for different uses in the facility and patients' care is crucial for work in any place and especially in PHC.

c. Communications: It is important to have at least two ways to contact the staff. If one method failed, the other will be the backup. A third wireless radio communication should be prepared for extreme loss of any sort of communication.

d. Network: Failure of network can occur alone or accompanying electricity failure. Server backup should be applied to keep the important information regarding patient, administrative, pharmacy, and store documents.

4.6 Stockpile stuff

During daily work, the PHC centers are stocking their expected needs of drugs and consumables for a certain period depending on the chain of supply. If there is a risk or threat of any type that needs special medications or protective equipment, the PHC centers should bring these stocks according to the population supported with the coordination of the local or national health authority.

5. Trans-impact phase

As mentioned above, the PHC will be the first point people will reach to seek help and advice regarding injuries or information regarding an epidemic infection. This includes many challenges.

5.1 Challenges

The WHO in their briefing about PHC and emergencies [9] mentioned some of the challenges as follows:

1. Without earlier warning system, case identification and escalation are a challenge that PHC staff face. Most epidemics usually start as patients come to seek medical advice, which is a day-to-day work in PHC. Case definition and raising the suspicion of a disease that may be an early epidemic or even pandemic (like the COVID-19) need to be reported to more central and higher authority with experts in epidemiology and infectious diseases.

2. Geographical accessibility:

    a. Several types of natural disasters like earthquake, floods, etc. may affect the PHC and its surrounding area, preventing health workers, people, or supply chain from reaching it. This will render the PHC useless, and alternative methods should be placed to mitigate this challenge.

    b. In the same context, geographical accessibility to patients and survivals will be sometimes difficult if not impossible and need special help.

    c. People with special need will face more difficulty in major incidents in accessing the PHC. The rescuers will face more difficulty in moving people with special needs in case there is need for it.

    d. Transferring patients and staff to an alternative place or transferring patients to hospital may be a challenge in certain circumstances.

3. Skillful health workers are part of the community and may be affected by the incidents either themselves or their families, and in both situations, they cannot be available to treat and help people. PHC may replace them by less skilled staff which will affect the care in this difficult situation.

4. Health facility infrastructure may be affected by the incident, and loss of water, electricity, and network supply, for example, will also affect the ability of PHC to offer help and services.

5. The incidents may affect the chain of supply, leading to a decrease in resources and limitations in the numbers and types of medications and services available.

6. If there is an incident that is big enough to affect large cities and states, the government will distribute the funds and resources to all areas. This mostly will make the amount given to a certain PHC center below its actual needs. This has effects on the availability of staff and supplements and decreases in the PHC center's effective services.

7. Ensuring quality of care to be in acceptable level. In day-to-day work, the quality should be in the optimum; this is not applicable in most MI, but there should be an agreed acceptable level of quality during major incident, so the PHC centers do not go below it. This is extremely important to decrease the spread of infectious diseases that follow major incidents and decrease mortality and morbidity for all patients.

5.2 Actions

There are many actions needed during the response phase. Those actions are classified according to the condition of the facility.

A. Health facility is intact, accessible, and functioning:

1. Activate the major incident response plan. This is the decision taken by PHC facility leader in liaison with the local and state health authority.

2. Change the layout of the facility and the patients' flow to permit faster management of patients with acceptable standards.

3. Call the staff who are in their off or vacation to join work in the facility to deal with the increased numbers of patients and visitors.

4. Stop elective visits of patients, and replace it by telephone or online consultations. If there is a need to see the patient and examine him physically, then go to him/her or call the patient to the center; examine the patient in area away from the incident management venue. This will decrease the number of patients attending to the health center and create surge capacity to examine patients related to the major incidents.

5. Contact local health authority and nearby hospitals to liaise about the situation and work distribution. The PHC can have an important role in dealing with the well and worried people and patients with mild symptoms to decrease the load on hospitals and minimize people's need for transportation. The movement restriction is an important factor in controlling epidemics and makes movement of emergency services easy and fast.

6. Make special documentation for the incident patients and other related issues like questionnaires, asking about relatives, etc. This will help in better preparedness for future incidents.

7. PHC director and supervisors should observe staff for signs of PTSD. Daily debriefing session should be done by the end of the shift. The management of PTSD staff will depend on the severity of symptoms.

    a. Mild PTSD usually is solved by the support of colleagues and the daily debriefing session.

    b. They may change the type or place of work of the staff if they noticed moderate symptoms of PTSD.

    c. Staff with severe symptoms of PTSD should be stopped from dealing with patients, and psychologist or psychiatrist consultation is requested.

B. If the primary health facility is not accessible or not functioning:

1. The alternative site should be activated, and directional signs to the new site, people, and authorities should be informed about the new site.

2. Medical teams [10, 11].

The concept of emergency medical teams applied in disaster management is well known worldwide and applied by the WHO and other bodies interested in disaster response. We can apply this concept to distribute the primary health staff into small teams and direct them (as forward teams) to different residential areas in conjunction with other emergency services. Their duty is to:

a. Define the special needs and vulnerable population.

b. Supply chronic medications to the needed.

c. Defining affected people and do baseline life support interventions.

d. Contact health authority or hospitals for patients who need to transfer to higher level of health care.

e. This concept, going to patients in their residency, can be used even if the facility is accessible and functioning. It is an extra service for people in catchment area aiming to bring health care very near to people and help in stopping the spread of epidemic infections.

C. Start thinking of recovery for the health centers during a long-lasting major incident, for example, the COVID-19 pandemic, which is affecting the whole world now. There should be regular thinking of how to resume work in the PHC to serve the patients who need regular follow-up. This can be done by telephone or network meeting (as mentioned above), and medications can be delivered to the patient at their homes through the post. Fees can be paid by electronic payment methods.

D. Live experience on the role of PHC in epidemic.

During the writing of this chapter, there is a COVID-19 epidemic. In the beginning of the epidemic, many people came to the emergency department asking for checkup and PCR test for COVID-19. This issue created overcrowding in emergency departments all over the country, and many people present are requesting the test. This was dangerous for spreading the infection if someone is really infected. Two days later, the PHC sets up centers for dealing with well and worried persons and provided COVID-19 PCR test. This action by the PHC did a huge decompression to emergency departments, decreased mix between well and feverish persons, and gave us opportunity to concentrate on symptomatic patients.

6. Post-impact phase

Recovery from the effects of the MI occurs in this phase. Sometimes, when the MI takes long time, the PHC should resume receiving patients other than MI. There is merging between trans-impact and post-impact phases. Recovery of the PHC will be better if it was part of the pre-incident plan [12].

6.1 Challenges

1. Many times, there are epidemics after major incidents especially if the incident affected the infrastructures of basic services like potable water and electricity. This effect is aggravated if people need to migrate from their area for any reason and

assemble in a new area, which is usually less suitable and overcrowded. This permits for disease transmission creating an epidemic between the migrants. Acute respiratory infections and cholera are among the most epidemics that occur in immigrants [13]. Some of these diseases are not present in the PHC area previously.

2. New patients may be added to the PHC from two sources:

   a. In the first source, there is an epidemic in the area covered by the PHC after the major incident. More patients are presented to PHC for consultations.

   b. The second source is the new people who moved to their area from other places, which rendered unsuitable for living (temporarily or permanently) by the major incident.

3. New diseases may occur due to loss of infrastructure and sanitation or due to earth changes, leading to bacterial, fungal, and other infectious organisms that are not common in the area. It is found in one study that there was an increase in visits for patients complaining of respiratory symptoms (mostly asthma) and diabetes [14].

4. In the last 40 years, all the studies showed that there is a significant increase in stress levels of both health care staffs and patients in post-major incident phase [15]. This will decrease the working staff on the one hand and increase the patients visiting the PHC on the other hand.

5. Delayed appointments for patients already registered in the PHC due to MI response actions. After the end of the incident, work need to be back to normal, and the patients whom appointments were postponed in the response period need to be rescheduled in addition to the regular appointments and providing appointments to the new patients.

6. Gathering information and statistics about the MI and its effects on the PHC in all aspects. Information regarding response to the major incidents, patients' flow, number of patients, types of complaints, areas of crowding and delay, etc. all need to be collected, summarized, studied, and used in this phase to prepare the PHC for improved response in the next major incident.

7. Funding. During the trans-impact phase, the media concentrate on every activity done by all emergency services. This media coverage is a good motivation for providing funds by governments, nongovernmental organizations, and personnel. In the post-impact phase, this media coverage will decrease a lot especially if there is another major incident in other parts of the world.

6.2 Actions

This stage is an opportunity to improve the PHC and rebuild it better than before, by applying risk reduction and optimizing work protocols [16]. The actions in the post-impact phase can be divided into three stages [17]:

a. Early recovery stage

   In this stage there is emphasis on clinical services; the PHC is trying to go back actively again. It is trying to open its services to people if the facility was closed during the incident's response phase or increase work if it was working in limited scope during the previous phase. The following are the steps to do this objective:

1. Maintain the PHC building, especially if it is affected by the incident. If there was an epidemic, then there is a need to deep cleaning and sterilization before allowing entrance and providing service to usual patients.

2. Debriefing to staff after the trans-impact phase. This may need psychologist or psychiatrist sometimes. The PHC director should evaluate the staff during all the phases. In this phase there is time to deal with the staff who shows mild-to-moderate PTSD.

3. Rearrange duty roasters for staff in a way that they can work and have time to look after their families.

4. Education to staff regarding new diseases that occurs in the post-impact phase. This should be arranged with local health authority and hospitals. There will be many questions regarding the new disease and relations to the chronic diseases they have.

b. Rehabilitation stage

The aim of this stage is to reach the pre-impact stage level of work and go back to normal activity or put a new norm to help in better response in the future. Activities in this stage are the following:

1. Maintain used equipment and fix the damaged ones. Electricity generators, water tanks, and ultrasound machines all should be checked by specialized teams.

2. Refill stores with medicines and consumables. When there is MI, there is large number of patients which is more than the present resources. After the end of the trans-impact phase, stores should be rearranged to have enough supply of the previous drugs and stuff for the new emerging diseases.

3. Rearrange patients' visits to decrease delay, and catch the condition before the incident.

4. Make appointments for the new patients added to the PHC facility after the impact. This may need recruitment of new staff to accommodate those patients in addition to the delayed patients mentioned in the previous point.

5. If an alternative place has been used and proven to be better than the original one, try using it permanently. All actions, official documentations, and addresses should be changed to the new place.

c. Development stage

This is a long-term stage, and its aim is to prepare the PHC for the next major incident. It will be mixed with the mitigation and preparedness stages in the pre-impact phase. To achieve this stage properly, there is a need to:

1. Collect data through statistics regarding different aspects of the incident, for example, numbers, diagnosis, age, etc.

2. Make plans for better facility; this may need change or an increase in facility building. Make plans to divide the facility into sectors if needed to maintain isolation for containing infections and easy sterilization of the parts of the facility. This should include the ventilation system of different areas.

3. Improve communication plan to the staff. All staff should have their contact addresses including the social media addresses and landlines if present.

4. Arrange with the local health authority to have any specific PHC plan to be part of a master plan and any PHC capabilities to add to the total state or national health abilities, and there is no need for doubling the work.

5. Fund raising should be started and requested from the local and state health authority to do all these changes in the facility and train the staff on different aspects of the MI response.

7. Conclusion

The primary health care system has big and important roles that can be played in response to major incidents. They are the most nearby health care facility and well known to people in each area, making it the nearest health facility that is ready to provide help when people are exposed to a sudden incident.

Their role is not limited to any stage in the incident, but it is in all phases. In some aspects of response, the primary health care staff will guide the state or national efforts to find and help vulnerable population in their catchment area.

More concentration on the primary health care system in terms of staff training, facility floor plans, and stuff stockpiling will yield a remarkable improvement in response to any major incidents.

Author details

Abdulnasir Falah Huaidi Al-Jazairi
FRCS (Glasgow), MScDM, Hamad Medical Corporation, Qatar

*Address all correspondence to: ahuaidi@hamad.qa

References

[1] Ray K, Ghimire J, Bc RK. Effects of disaster on primary health care in low income countries. Journal of Nepal Health Research Council. 2019;**17**(1): 1-8. DOI: 10.33314/jnhrc.1688

[2] Park S, Abrams R. Alma-Ata 40th birthday celebrations and the Astana declaration on primary health care 2018. The British Journal of General Practice. 2019;**69**(682):220-221

[3] Sheiham A. Closing the gap in a generation: Health equity through action on the social determinants of health. A report of the WHO Commission on social determinants of health (CSDH) 2008. Community Dental Health. 2009;**26**(1):2-3

[4] World Health Organization. Primary health care. 2019. Available from: https://www.who.int/news-room/fact-sheets/detail/primary-health-care [Accessed: 28 February 2020]

[5] Comprehensive Care, Definition of AAFP. Available from: https://www.aafp.org/about/policies/all/care-definition.html [Accessed: 22 March 2020]

[6] Available from: http://www.mimms.org.au/major-incidents [Accessed: 22 March 2020]

[7] Waisel DB. Vulnerable populations in healthcare. Current Opinion in Anaesthesiology. 2013;**26**(2):186-192

[8] Rodriguez H, Quarantelli EL, Dynes RR. Handbook of Disaster Research. Switzerland: Springer; 2007

[9] "Primary Health care and Health Emergencies." World Health Organization. Available from: https://apps.who.int/iris/rest/bitstreams/1251548/retrieve [Accessed: 24 March 2020]

[10] Norton I, et al. Available from: Www.who.int, www.who.int/hac/global_health_cluster/fmt_guidelines_september2013.pdf [Accessed: 26 March 2020]

[11] Reis ND, Dolev E. Manual of Disaster Medicine: Civilian and Military. Berlin: Springer-Verlag; 1989 [Accessed: 27 March 2020]

[12] Cometto G, Fritsche G, Sondorp E. Health sector recovery in early post-conflict environments: Experience from southern Sudan. Disasters. 2010;**34**(4):885-909 [Accessed: 27 March 2020]

[13] Watson JT, Gayer M, Connolly MA. Epidemics after natural disasters. Emerging Infectious Diseases. 2007;**13**(1):1-5. DOI: 10.3201/eid1301.060779 [Accessed: 28 March 2020]

[14] Chowdhury MAB, Fiore AJ, Cohen SA, et al. Health impact of hurricanes Irma and Maria on St Thomas and St John, US Virgin Islands, 2017-2018. American Journal of Public Health. 2019;**109**(12):1725-1732. DOI: 10.2105/AJPH.2019.305310 [Accessed: 28 March 2020]

[15] Galea S, Nandi A, Vlahov D. The epidemiology of post-traumatic stress disorder after disasters. Epidemiologic Reviews. 2005;**27**(1):78-91. DOI: 10.1093/epirev/mxi003 [Accessed: 28 March 2020]

[16] Mortlock A, Vasconez AC, Bittner P, Alatrista CB, Matsuoka Y. Disaster Recovery Guidance Series: Health Sector Recovery - World. ReliefWeb. 2017. Available from: https://reliefweb.int/report/world/disaster-recovery-guidance-series-health-sector-recovery [Accessed: 27 March 2020]

[17] Al-Jazairi A. Disasters and disaster medicine. In: Alsheikhly AS, editor. Essentials of Accident and Emergency Medicine. UK: BoD – Books on Demand; 2019. pp. 111-112. DOI: 10.5772/intechopen.71634

Chapter 7

Pharmacoeconomical Impacts of Crohn's Disease

Stjepan Rudan, Rudika Gmajnić and Sanda Pribić

Abstract

Provide an overview of Crohn's disease and its cost assessment options, establish the need for implementing Croatian national Crohn's Disease Registry to precisely quantify the costs and the outcomes, and establish model to evaluate values of treatment options for Crohn's disease.

Keywords: Crohn's disease, farmacoeconomical impact

1. Introduction

Crohn's disease is a chronic, progressive inflammatory bowel disease (IBD). Although mortality is rare, Crohn's disease significantly impacts quality of life as it causes significant disabilities related to the debilitating symptoms and complications of the disease and its treatment. As such, IBD exerts physical, social, sexual, emotional, educational, and job-related limitations. Therefore Crohn's disease produces a huge burden on patients, families, and societies.

While it is clear that new biological therapies have raised the bar for what is an acceptable symptomatic response in Crohn's disease, the key pharmacoeconomical and humanical questions are whether TNF antagonists can reduce hospitalization and surgery rates or can, if applied in earlier stages, modify the course of the disease by means of fistula healing, mucosal healing, and overall improvement in QOL [1].

Novel therapies and alternative treatment algorithms require that healthcare providers evaluate the value of these treatments. Pharmacoeconomic analyses aim to assess whether new technologies are superior to existing treatments by relating costs to outcomes.

In the absence of the national registry, in Croatia, we do not have national data on Crohn's disease; therefore in this paper, we can only apply epidemiological models to project Crohn's disease costs and pharmacoeconomically evaluate treatment options.

2. How to evaluate CD therapies: clinical indexes and endpoints

Traditional primary endpoints in clinical trials (i.e., Crohn's Disease Activity Index (CDAI)) quantify physical symptoms, without incorporating overall "illness experience."

Therefore, QOL measures are commonly used as secondary endpoints in clinical trials, and several QOL tools are available. Since the first being created in 1985, the development of IBD questionnaires has substantially advanced studies of HRQOL. In addition to the common physical complaints associated with CD, IBDQ also measures social, functional, and psychological factors, and it has strong correlation to CD (Shah 1). A total of 32 items comprise the questionnaire, being grouped into 4 major domains (bowel function, social function, emotional functional, and systemic function). Total score ranges from 32 to 224 points, higher score indicating better QOL (Shah 2). Several validation studies of IBDQ were performed in different populations confirming its validity (Shah 3). A score above 170 is considered desirable [2–4].

To better address patient concerns in regard to the effects of the disease and their health status, rating form of IBD patient concerns was developed [5].

However, review study assessing several HRQOL tools led to the conclusion that IBDQ was simple, reliable, and accurate in disease activity assessment and therefore more favorable than other instruments [6].

3. Medical treatments: outcomes

Corticosteroids have long been used in the management of Crohn's disease. They demonstrate rapid onset of action and efficacy while having significant side effect profile and lack of maintenance benefit [7]. The need for corticosteroids' use is a significant indicator of future disabling disease and complications, including mortality [8, 9]. One analysis has shown that Crohn's disease patients using corticosteroids had 38% risk for surgery in 1 year [10].

While it is clear that new biological therapies have raised the bar for what is an acceptable symptomatic response in Crohn's disease, the key pharmacoeconomical and humanical questions are whether TNF antagonists can reduce hospitalization and surgery rates or can, if applied in earlier stages, modify the course of the disease by means of fistula healing, mucosal healing, and overall improvement in QOL.

ACCENT I trial has clearly demonstrated efficacy of infliximab maintenance treatment in patients with fistulizing Crohn's disease [11]. Further subgroup analysis has shown that in patients randomized to maintenance infliximab treatment following successfully induction therapy, the mean number of hospital days per 100 patients treated was significantly reduced in the group of patients assigned to infliximab compared with those who received placebo [12]. Significant reductions in the rates of surgery and procedures were also demonstrated [12].

CHARM trial [13] confirmed adalimumab efficacy and safety in moderate to severe Crohn's disease. Based on CHARM data, the effect of ongoing adalimumab treatment on the risk for hospitalization was evaluated [14]. It showed a significant difference between placebo and adalimumab group, demonstrating relative risk reduction of 57% and absolute risk reduction 8%, showing the difference between the treatment groups early in the course of the therapy. Multivariable analysis confirmed that assignment to adalimumab therapy was inversely correlated with the risk of hospitalization and surgery.

These studies confirmed that TNF antagonists can reduce the risk of hospitalization and surgery in Crohn's disease. Together with Lemann trial on infliximab [15], both trials confirmed that anti-TNF agents are effective steroid-sparing agents.

In the provocative trial inverting the treatment pyramid [16], newly diagnosed patients with symptomatic disease were randomized either to infliximab + azathioprine combination (top-down group) or to steroids initially (step-up group), which were increased if patients flared during taper, or azathioprine and a second course of steroids if patients flared after the initial steroid course was completed. If symptoms recurred, or the response was inadequate, infliximab was given. Remission of steroids without surgery was achieved in 60% of patients in top-down group vs. 36% of patients in step-up group at 26 weeks and 62% vs. 42% of the patients, respectively, at 56 weeks.

As approximately one third of the patients with Crohn's disease will develop fistulas at some point in the disease course [17], it is important to underline that both infliximab [18] and adalimumab [13] were proven effective for the partial or complete healing of fistulas in patients with Crohn's disease, maintaining the effect among responders in majority of patients at 1 year.

Mucosal healing as a potential disease-modifying point was reported superior in patients receiving infliximab in an endoscopic sub study of the ACCENT I trial [19]. This is even more important knowing that mucosal healing findings have not correlated well with clinical remission by CDAI: 56% of patients in remission by CDAI did not have mucosal healing. The reasons for this remain unclear.

In a sub study of step-up was top-down trial [20], 44 patients were endoscopically evaluated at year 2 from initiation of the treatment, and results were compared with endoscopy findings at the diagnosis. For the comparison, five ileal and colonic segment lesions were scored for each patient. Complete ulcer disappearance was observed in 71% of patients who received top-down vs. 30% of patients who received step-up treatment. Mucosal healing was more pronounced in top-down group, with ulcer reductions observed in 88% of patients in top-down vs. 47% of patients in step-up group. The results indicate that infliximab is effective for the induction of mucosal healing. Effects of adalimumab have not been reported.

Finally, both infliximab and adalimumab were associated with improvements in QOL scores:

ACCENT I studied HRQOL [21], suggesting substantial impairment HRQOL at baseline scores and substantial improvements throughout the infliximab maintenance therapy.

CLASSIC II trial [22] demonstrated that patients on maintenance adalimumab therapy achieving remission have demonstrated improvements in IBDQ that were maintained throughout 1 year.

It can be concluded that both infliximab and adalimumab are significantly more effective in improving both CDAI and HRQOL than other treatment options. Also, it is suggested that reverting the treatment algorithm and introducing infliximab earlier on (top-down approach) may result in better mucosal healing and therefore modify the course of the disease.

4. Costs of the disease

Crohn's disease patients are typically diagnosed at their young age, and the treatment is generally lifelong.

Patients require chronic drug therapy due to the recurrent episodes of abdominal pain, diarrhea, and bleeding. Conventional therapies (glucocorticoids and immunosuppressives) are effective but associated with considerable side effects. Biological therapies have been introduced into routine clinical use, improving the disease outcomes over the past decade [11–14]; however, the costs related to novel options are substantially higher.

Hospitalization and surgeries are often needed to manage complications such as abscesses, perforations, and obstructions. Bowel resections are associated with considerable morbidity and, infrequently, death.

It is clear that both symptoms and the treatment of Crohn's disease reduce patients' health-related quality of life (HRQOL).

Cost of illness studies has showed that hospitalization and surgery are major factors of the total societal costs of Crohn's disease [23–25].

But above these obvious disease management costs, work loss and impaired HRQOL increase the humanistic and economic burden in Crohn's disease.

4.1 Direct costs: disease management costs—course and prognosis related

Direct costs are easily identifiable and quantifiable. The costs of Crohn's disease include outpatient care costs (medications, tests, procedures) and inpatient care costs (hospitalization).

In a prospective study [26], 33% of patients with chronic or intermittently active disease required hospitalization and surgery after developing complications in the first year following diagnosis, and 13% required hospitalization and surgery in the second year and 3% in each following year.

The same study showed that 20% of CD patients were unable to work at full capacity 20 years after the time of diagnosis. Another long-term follow-up study showed that approximately 74% of all patients with CD will eventually be hospitalized and ultimately require surgical intervention for their disease [27].

4.2 Indirect costs: total economic loss experienced by patients, caregivers, and society/HRQOL-related costs

Indirect costs are more subjective than direct costs. In Crohn's disease, sources of indirect costs include absence from work, premature retirement, and the social and psychological effects of chronic disease on patients and their families.

As a consequence of the Crohn's disease course and prognosis, HRQOL is diminished and directly correlates with a higher likelihood of unemployment [28]. In a case-controlled study [29], adult patients with CD were reported to have more long-term unemployment than controls. Furthermore, in the same study, up to 30% of CD patients were reported to concealed their illness from their employers.

As determined in ACCENT I [30], there were high unemployment rates of 27% in males and 44% in females among Crohn's disease patients. However, only 25% of patients received disability benefits. This further strengthens economic burden of Crohn's disease to society.

5. How to evaluate CD therapies: costs vs. outcomes

As societal resources for healthcare are limited, sound methodology for resource allocation is needed. Pharmacoeconomic analyses address this issue, considering costs (currency) and the consequences of the therapy. In 2007 Feagan [31] posted an effective overview of the methodology, commonly classified into four categories: cost-minimization, cost-effectiveness, cost–benefit, and cost-utility analyses. The differences between methodologies are based on the outcome to which costs are related.

When two competing interventions have equivalent clinical outcomes, it is logical to use *Cost-minimization analysis*. Being the most simple analysis, it favors less costly treatment when no clinical difference has been demonstrated.

In more often, real-life cases, when we are faced with new therapies that are both more effective and more expensive, we have to relate different costs and different outcomes. Therefore other more sophisticated methodologies are needed [32].

Cost-effectiveness analysis relates costs to clinically meaningful differences in outcomes: per beneficial outcome attained, the incremental cost of a novel therapy is then expressed in terms of currency expended. It can be used in indications where robust endpoints exist (i.e., myocardial infarction prevention) and the incremental costs are easily understood by patients and providers [32].

Cost-benefit analysis translates differences in outcomes into monetary terms, as they are for the costs. This brings two inputs into the same units, and the comparison between the treatments is easily interpreted. Logically, the strategy that maximizes net value for the society (net currency gained) is preferred. Relevance of this technique in terms of healthcare applicability is challenged: it requires value judgments, which are usually inappropriate [33].

Cost-utility analysis expresses currency expended per incremental improvement in HRQOL achieved. It evaluates well chronic diseases with serious impact on HRQOL, but without causing excess mortality or frequent complications. The HRQOL measure used is utility. This is a generic metric placing a value on HRQOL, ranging from 1 (perfect health) to 0 (death). Quality-adjusted life years (QALYs) are then derived by multiplying the time in a health state by the appropriate utility score. Logically, differences between treatments are expressed as the incremental costs per QALY gained [34].

Cost of illness studies identify where efficacies can be realized. These studies are descriptive evaluations that (1) assess the total economic burden of the disease; (2) define the relative proportions of total costs allocated to diagnostic tests, healthcare professionals, institutions, and drugs; and (3) generate hypotheses regarding the economic consequences of treatment alternatives.

Only a few such studies have been reported for Crohn's disease.

A cost model for IBD was created in the early 1990s using data from a California health maintenance organization [23]. Reducing the charges obtained from a teaching hospital in San Francisco by 35%, the mean annual medical cost of Crohn's disease was estimated to be 6561$ per person. It was demonstrated that approximately 20% of patients generate 80% of healthcare costs. Surgery and hospitalization were associated with 79.9% of the average costs of medical services. Drug therapy was responsible for 10.2% of the total costs. By extrapolating these data to the US population, using published prevalence estimates and 1990 census data, the total direct cost of Crohn's disease was estimated to be 1–1.2 billion annually, compared to 0.4–0.6 billion for ulcerative colitis. The indirect costs of the disease were estimated based exclusively on lost labor productivity and calculated 0.4–0.8 billion annually. Therefore, the total (direct + indirect) economic burden for IBD (Crohn and UC) was estimated to be 1.8–2.6 bio $ yearly [23].

Feagan's study [24] evaluated reimbursement charges from patients enrolled in a health benefit claims program serving 50 largest US employers. Eligible patients were enrolled in their health plan for a minimum of 3 years and had at least 1 CD-related claim over a 1-year interval (1994/1995). The study retrospectively classified patients into three mutually exclusive status: mild (patients in remission or those requiring less than 6 months of active treatment during the observation period), moderate (patients who required chronic treatment for more than 6 months with prednisone or antimetabolites), and severe disease (patients requiring admission to hospital for treatment). A total of 607 patients generated average annual charges of 12.417$ per patient: 6.277$ being the average for the mild, 10.033$ for the moderate, and 37.135$ for the severe form of the disease.

These studies suggest that treatments that reduce the need for hospitalization or surgery may result in important cost savings.

As quoted earlier on, two subgroups of large randomized clinical trials have strongly indicated that the use of TNF antagonists reduces the rate of hospitalization and surgery in Crohn's disease [12, 14].

It is important to evaluate in economic models whether the potential offsets that result from reduced rates of hospitalization and surgery justify the high price of biological.

Lindsay et al. [35] used Markov models to simulate the disease progression and track associated costs and outcomes as QALYs over 5 years of treatment in hypothetical cohort of patients with active luminal or fistulizing CD, during treatment with infliximab (5 mg/kg). Transitions were estimated from published clinical trials of infliximab. Standard care, comprising immunomodulators, and seven corticosteroids were used as a comparator. An average weight of 60 kg was used to estimate the dose of infliximab. Authors discounted the costs and outcomes 3.5% over 5 years. The primary effectiveness measurement was quality-adjusted life years estimated using EQ-5D. One-way and probabilistic sensitivity analyses were used by varying infliximab efficacy estimates, costs, and utilities. The incremental costs per QALY gained were 26.128P in luminal and 29.752 in fistulizing CD at 5 years. Results were robust, remaining in the range of 23.752–38.848 for luminal and 27.047–44.206 for fistulizing CD. Not surprisingly, the most important factor affecting cost-effectiveness was patients' body weight. The authors concluded that 8-week scheduled maintenance treatment with infliximab is a cost-effective treatment for adult patients suffering from active luminal or fistulizing CD.

6. Where we are in Croatia and how we should move forward

In Croatia there is no national registry of Crohn's disease. Therefore, we are lacking precise epidemiological data that are essential for high-quality cost-utility/ HRQOL assessments.

Consequently, we do not have exact data on the total incidence and prevalence of the disease. We cannot precisely conclude how many of Croatian patients are suffering from the mild, moderate, or severe form of the disease. We also cannot confirm precise age or weight distribution of the patients. We also do not know the educational distribution or the rate of unemployment among Crohn's disease patients.

As it concerns outpatient care costs, while we can find IMS data or HZZO data on total cost of biological therapies, we do not have the access to cost split per indication. Also we are not aware on how much resources are allocated to other outpatient care elements.

Furthermore, we cannot define essential resource allocation inputs for Crohn's disease. There is no available source to confirm the exact number of hospital days/ related costs due to Crohn's disease or to provide exact number of surgery procedures/related costs undertaken for Crohn's disease. We do not know how much is spent on side effect management. Also we cannot define the disease costs per mild, moderate, and severe form of the disease.

Related to the lack of the national registry, we cannot quantify DASS and IBDQ improvements related to treatments applied; therefore we cannot define price per HRQOL improvement.

What we can do at this point is to improvise: to extrapolate epidemiological data [36, 37] and estimate the incidence and the prevalence of the disease in Croatia. Then we can apply international data to estimate patients' split and treatment outcomes and average cost per patient group. Then we can use Markov models and analyses as implemented by Lindsay et al. [35].

The above mentioned leaves calculation table empty at basic input level. Our first conclusion is that there is an essential need to implement national IBD registry to summarize the data needed for an economic analysis model.

Our second conclusion taken from CD example is that if we want to better drive our HC resources, *Cost-effectiveness analysis* needs to become the key method for assessing costs and benefits of alternative ways of allocating resources to assist decisions aiming to improve efficiency. An efficient allocation of resources implies that no further health gains can be achieved by allocating the same resources differently. The analysis is based on maximizing health effects subject to a cost constraint, where costs are measured in monetary units and health effects in non-monetary units, such as life years or quality-adjusted life years. QALYs are constructed by adjusting life years for the quality of life in which they are spent. To achieve this, the number of years in a health state is multiplied by utility weight between 0 (dead) and 1 (full health). To determine whether a treatment is cost-effective compared to alternative, the cost per gained unit of effectiveness (i.e., cost per QALY gained) must be compared with the willingness to pay (WTP) for a gained unit of effectiveness (i.e., the value of QALY gained). WTP can be defined as the price the payer is willing to pay for a QALY. If the price per unit increase in effectiveness exceeds the target price, then the program is cost-effective. Without the information about the price per unit increase in effectiveness, CEA gives no information on whether an intervention is cost-effective. The value of a QALY differs between courtiers and is logically related to the level of GDP.

7. CD example/Markov models: how to implement it in Croatia

The model characterizes the disease severity by two discrete "on-treatment" health states: (1) remission (DAI </=150) and (2) response but no remission/active state (CDAI >150). All patients started in the active state and remained as such for the first model cycle. At the end of the first and each subsequent model cycle, patients either remained in the active state or moved to a different health state. In the illustration of the model bellow, two separate numbers denote different transitions in standard care and infliximab* treatment arm. If single number, there were no differences between the arms.

Patients responding to treatment and achieving CDAI </= 150 moved to the remission and remained on treatment. Patients responding but not achieving remission remained in the active state and continued treatment [11]. Nonresponders or discontinuing-from-treatment patients moved to the nonresponding active state. Once patients failed the treatment and discontinued from the treatment, they could not go back to the on-treatment status, but they were followed up to capture costs and outcomes.

As obvious from diagrams, both on-treatment and off-treatment patients could transition to surgery. Following surgery, patients could either undergo repeat surgery due to immediate complications, therefore remaining in surgery state, or they could move to a post surgery health state (remission or post surgery complications). Patients in post surgery remission could continue in the same health state, enter surgery for repeated procedure, enter post surgery complication state, or have CD recurrence and move to a nonresponsive active state. Infliximab failures were not re-treated, and also patients with post surgery complications could continue in the same health state, enter surgery, respond to treatment for their complications and enter post surgery remission, or have recurrence of CD and enter nonresponding active state.

In model adjusted for fistulizing DC, on-treatment health states of remission were further sub classified as with or without failure. This gives four on-treatment health states as shown in the diagram. The rest of the model was identical to the active luminal CD model.

The patient and treatment parameters (sources of efficacy estimation, treatment regimen, comparators, treatment strategy) in Markov models are based on standard treatment protocols and ACCENT trial evidence [11, 18]. Treatment horizon was 5 years.

Before establishing national registry, as suggested in Lindsay trial [35], transition probabilities for different health states could be taken from published randomized placebo-controlled induction studies [38].

Consequently, before establishing the national registry, probability of surgery, postsurgical states, and CD recurrence are to be obtained from the literature [39–44].

Costs resulting from the impact of CD on QOL and productivity and overall burden to the Croatian society are difficult to estimate based on international trial findings [45, 46] and might be disregarded at this initial point of establishing CEA model.

Drug costs per indication are drug acquisition costs (price per pack), drug administration costs (price per infusion in the case of infliximab), and price of concomitant drugs (immunomodulators, aminosalisylates, corticosteroids).

These drug costs can be obtained from HZZO or from the national CD registry.

Alternatively we can calculate drug acquisition costs assuming an average body weight of 60 kg based on NICE guidance for infliximab case.

Surgery, hospitalization, and other assessment costs should be obtained from HZZO [47].

The primary efficacy measure of Croatian CD model should be QALY, gains being driven by quality-of-life benefits. Utility as a measure places a value on HRQOL, ranging from 1 (perfect health) to 0 (death). Quality-adjusted life years are then derived by multiplying the time in a health state by the appropriate utility score. Cost-utility analysis represents incremental cost per QALY gained. Logically, differences between treatments should be expressed as the differences in incremental costs per QALY. Cost and outcomes are to be calculated in accordance with NICE guidelines, separately for the entire cohort of patients in treatment arms, regardless of their response rates, and discounted to present values at 3.5% per annum.

7.1 Markov model for active luminal CD

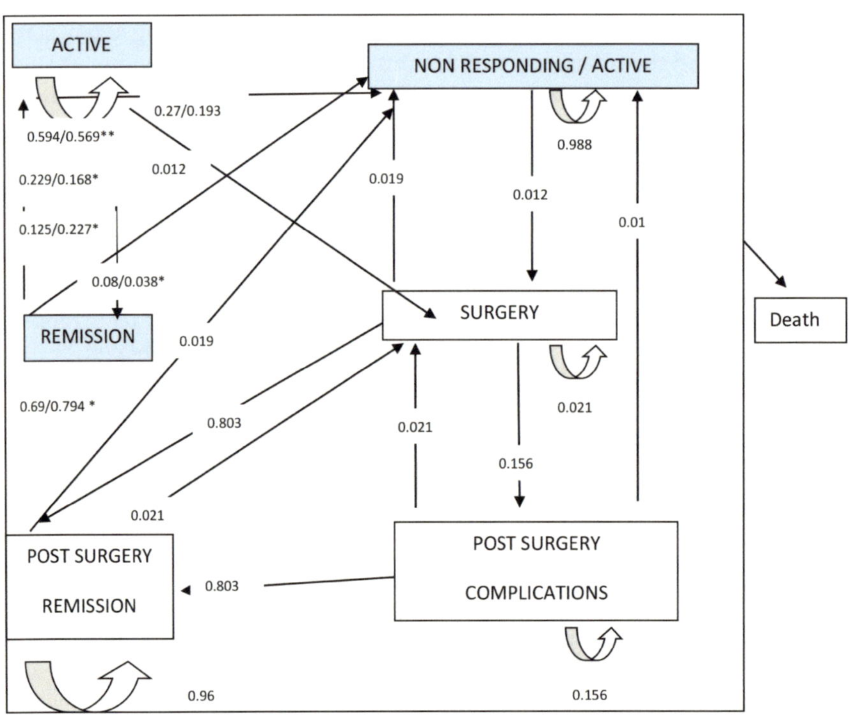

7.2 Markov model modified for fistulizing CD

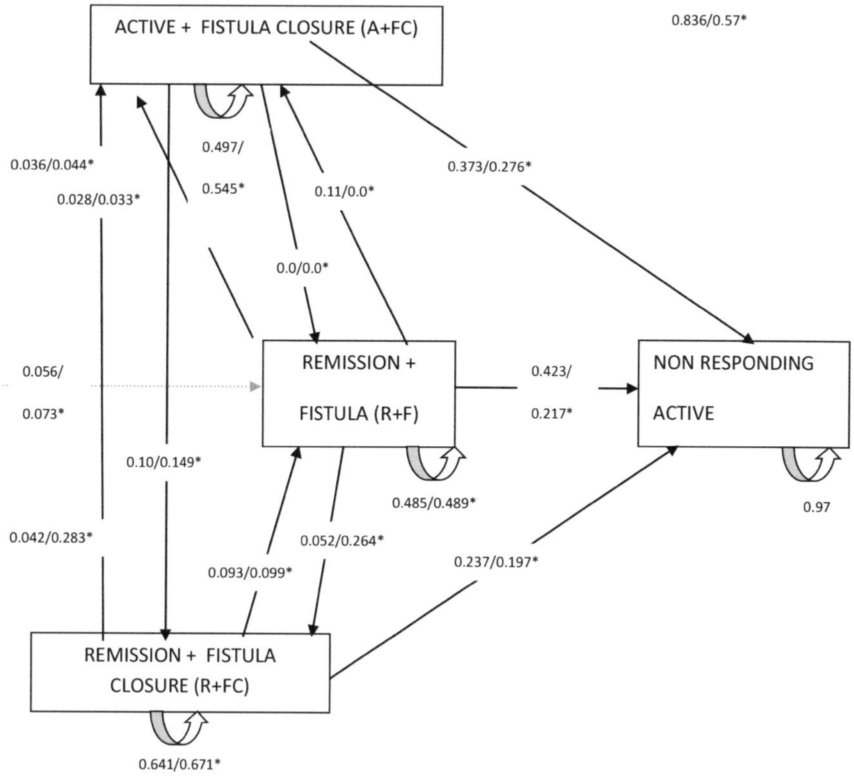

8. Conclusions

Based on international trials, TNF antagonists' maintenance therapy may bring significant improvements in patients' HRQOL in adult patients with severe active luminal or fistulizing CD.

Based on international cost-utility analyses, it can be concluded that a substantial part of TNF antagonist acquisition costs could be offset by savings on other disease-related costs in patients not responding to or intolerant to steroids and immunomodulators.

It is essential to establish Croatian National Registry of Crohn's disease to prospectively evaluate epidemiology, clinical subgroups, transition from states, treatment outcomes, and costs.

Markov models combined with registry data and findings from international trials represent solid frame to calculate pharmacoeconomic impacts of Crohn's disease treatments.

From the payers perspective, it seems to be a must to establish a QALY-based process of assessment of new therapeutic options and HC technologies in Croatia. Using this methodology, payers would develop comparable data even in different indications/treatment options, evaluate objectively contributions for incremental costs per QALY, and allocate HR resources accordingly.

Author details

Stjepan Rudan[1], Rudika Gmajnić[2,3]* and Sanda Pribić[1,3]

1 Faculty of Dental Medicine and Health Osijek, Croatia

2 Medical Faculty of Osijek, Croatia

3 European University Brčko District, Bosnia and Herzegovina

*Address all correspondence to: rudika.gmajnic01@gmail.com

References

[1] Velayos UM. Medscape Gastroenterology [Medscape]. 2008. [Posted: 03/18/2008]

[2] Kirshner B, Guyat G. A methodological framework for assessing health indices. Journal of Chronic Diseases. 1985;**38**:27-36

[3] Guyat G, Mitchell A, Irvine EJ, et al. A new measure of health status for clinical trials in inflammatory bowel disease. Gastroenterology. 1989;**96**:804-810

[4] Irvine EJ, Feagan B, Rochon J, et al. Quality of life: A valid and reliable measure of therapeutic efficacy in the treatment of inflammatory bowel disease. Canadian Crohn's relapse prevention trial study group. Gastroenterology. 1994;**106**:287-296

[5] Drossman DA, Leserman J, Li ZM, et al. The rating from IBD patient concerns: A new measure of health status. Psychosomatic Medicine. 1991;**53**:701-712

[6] Pallis AG, Mouzas IA. Instruments for quality of life assessment in patients with gastrointestinal cancer. Anticancer Research. 2004;**24**:2117-2121

[7] Summers RW, Switz DM, Sessions JT Jr, et al. National cooperative Crohn's disease study: Results of drug treatment. Gastroenterology. 1979;**77**:847-869

[8] Beaugerie L, Sesik P, Nion-Larmurier I, et al. Predictors of Crohn's disease. Gastroenterology. 2006;**130**:650-656

[9] Lichtenstein GR, Feagan BG, Cohen RD, et al. Serious infections and mortality in association with therapies for Crohn's disease: TREAT registry. Clinical Gastroenterology and Hepatology. 2006;**4**:621-630

[10] Faubion WA Jr, Loftus EV Jr, Hamsen WS, et al. The natural history of corticosteroid therapy for inflammatory bowel disease: A population based study. Gastroenterology. 2001;**121**:255-260

[11] Hanauer SB, Feagan BG, Lichtenstein GR, et al. Maintenance infliximab for Crohn's disease: The ACCENT I randomised trial. Lancet. 2002;**359**:1541-1549

[12] Lichtenstein GR, Yan S, Bala M, et al. Infliximab maintenance treatment reduces hospitalizations, surgeries and procedures in fistulizing Crohn's disease. Gastroenterology. 2005;**128**:862-869

[13] Colombel JF, Sandborn WJ, Rutgeerts P, et al. Adalimumab for maintenance of clinical response and remission in patients with Crohn's disease: The CHARM trial. Gastroenterology. 2007;**132**:52-65

[14] Feagan BG, Panaccione R, Sandborn W, et al. An evaluation of adalimumab on the risk of hospitalization in patients with Crohn's disease, data from CHARM. Gastroenterology. 2007;**132**:A-513/T1312

[15] Leman M, Mary JY, Duclos B, et al. Infliximab plus azathioprine for steroid dependent Crohn's disease patients: A randomized placebo –controlled trial. Gastroenterology. 2006;**130**:1054-1061

[16] D'Haens G, Baert F, van Assche G, et al. Early combined immunosuppression or conventional management in patients with newly diagnosed Crohn's disease: An open randomized trial. Lancet. 2008;**371**:660-667

[17] Schwartz DA, Loftus EV Jr, Tremaine WJ, et al. The natural history of fistulizing Crohn's disease in Olmsted country, Minnesota. Gastroenterology. 2002;**122**:875-880

[18] Sands BE, Anderson FH, Bernstein CN, et al. Infliximab maintenance therapy for fistulizing Crohn's disease. The New England Journal of Medicine. 2004;**350**:228-238

[19] Ruetgers P, Diamond R, Bala M, et al. Scheduled maintenance treatment with infliximab is superior to episodic treatment for the healing of mucosal ulceration associated with Crohn's disease. Gastrointestinal Endoscopy. 2006;**63**:433-442. quiz 464

[20] D'Haens GHD, Baert F, et al. A combined regimen of infliximab and azathioprine induces better endoscopic healing than classic step up therapy in newly diagnosed Crohn's disease. Gastroenterology. 2006;**130**:A-110

[21] Feagan BG, Yan S, Bala M, et al. The effects of infliximab maintenance therapy on health related quality of life. The American Journal of Gastroenterology. 2003;**98**:2232-2238

[22] Ruetgeerts PML, Li J, et al. Adalimumab maintains improvement in inflammatory bowel disease questionnaire (IBDQ) scores over 1 year following the initial attainment of remission in patients with moderately to severe active Crohn's disease. Gastroenterology. 2006;**130**:A-479

[23] Hay JW, Hay AR. Inflammatory bowel disease. Cost of illness. Journal of Clinical Gastroenterology. 1992;**14**:309-317

[24] Feagan BG, Larson LR VMG, Bala MV. Annual cost of care for Crohn's disease: A payor perspective. The American Journal of Gastroenterology. 2000;**95**:1955-1960

[25] Silversteing MD, Loftus EV, Sandborn WJ, et al. Clinical course and costs of care for Crohn's disease: Markov model analysis of a population based cohort. Gastroenterology. 1999;**117**:49-57

[26] Binder V, Hendriksen C, Kreiner S. Prognosis in Crohn's disease—Based on results from a regional patient group from the county of Copenhagen. Gut. 1985;**26**:146-150

[27] Farmer RG, Whelan G, Fazio VW. Long term follow up of patients with Crohn's disease. Relationship between the clinical pattern and prognosis. Gastroenterology. 1985;**88**:1818-1825

[28] Zisma TL, Cohen RD. Pharmacoeconomics and quality of life of current and emerging biologic therapies for inflammatory bowel disease. Current Treatment Options in Gastroenterology. 2007;**10**:185-194

[29] Mayberry MK, Probert C, Srivastava E, et al. Perceived discrimination in education and employment by people with Crohn's disease: A case control study of educational achievement and employment. Gut. 1992;**33**:312-214

[30] Feagan BG, Bala M, Yan S, et al. Unemployment and disability in patients with moderately to severe active Crohn's disease. Journal of Clinical Gastroenterology. 2005;**39**:390-395

[31] Feagan BG. The economics of Crohn's disease: TNF agonists and the impact of prevention and hospitalization. Medscape Gastroenterology. 2007. Medscape Posted 06719/2007

[32] Rittenhouse B. Designing and conducting cost minimization and cost-effectiveness analyses. In: Spilker B, editor. Quality of Life and Pharmacoeconomics in Clinical Trials. Philadelphia: Lippincot Raven; 1996. pp. 1093-1103

[33] Johannesson M, Weinstein MC. Designing and conducting cost benefit analysis. In: Spilker B, editor. Quality of Life and Pharmacoeconomics in Clinical Trials. Philadelphia: Lippincot Raven; 1996. pp. 1085-1092

[34] Torrance G. Designing and conducting cost utility analysis. In: Spilker B, editor. Quality of Life and Pharmacoeconomics in Clinical Trials. Philadelphia: Lippincot Raven; 1996. pp. 1105-1111

[35] Lindsay J, Punekar YS, Morris J, et al. Health economic analysis: Cost effectiveness of scheduled maintenance treatment with infliximab for Crohn's disease—Modelling outcomes in active luminal and fistulizing disease in adults. Alimentary Pharmacology & Therapeutics. 2008;**28**:1230-1239

[36] Sincic Mijandrusic B, Vucelic B, Persic M et al. Incidence of IBD in Primorsko Goranska County, Croatia 2000-2004: A prospective population based study

[37] Vrhovac B et al. Internal Medicine. 1991

[38] Present DH, Rutgeerts P, Targan S, et al. Infliximab for the treatment of fistulas in patients with Crohn's disease. The New England Journal of Medicine. 1999;**340**:1398-1405

[39] Munkolm P, Langholz E, Davidsen M, Binder V. Intestinal cancer risk and mortality in patients with Crohn's disease. Gastroenterology. 1993;**105**:1716-1723

[40] Cosnes J, Nion-Larmurier I, Beaugerie L, et al. Impact of the increasing use of immunosuppressants in Crohn's disease on the need for intestinal surgery. Gut. 2005;**54**:237-241

[41] Jess T, Loftus E, Scot Harmsen W, et al. Survival and cause specific mortality in patients with IBD: A long term outcome study in Olmsted country, Minnesota 1940-2004. Gut. 2006;**55**:1248-1255

[42] Marchal L, D'haens G, Van Assche G, et al. The risk of postoperative complications associated with infliximab therapy for Crohn's disease: A controlled cohort study. Alimentary Pharmacology & Therapeutics. 2004;**19**:749-754

[43] Fl W, Russel MG, Sijbrandij J, et al. Phenotype at diagnosis predicts recurrence rates in CD. Gut. 2006;**55**:1124-1130

[44] Makowiec F, Jehle EC, Starlinger M. Clinical course of perianal fistulas in CD. Gut. 1995;**37**:696-701

[45] Munkolm P, Langholz E, Davidsen M, Binder V. Disease activity courses in a regional cohort of Crohn's disease patients. Scandinavian Journal of Gastroenterology. 1995;**30**:699-706

[46] Hanauer SB, Cohen RD, Becker RV, et al. Advances in the management of Crohn's disease: Economic and clinical potential of infliximab. Clinical Therapeutics. 1998;**20**:1009-1028

[47] Bassi A, Dodd S, Williamson P, Bodger K. Cost of illness of inflammatory bowel disease in the UK. A single Centre retrospective study. Gut. 2004;**53**:1471-1478

Chapter 8

Visual Pathologies: The Semiotics of the Patient and the Practitioner in Comics

Jonathan Comyn de Rothewelle

Abstract

Newspapers have been a stronghold news source for centuries covering a wide range of topics. Though reporting is meant to be unbiased and only fact, stories produced are inevitably entwined with the author's cultural values—news content ranging from sports to healthcare, including articles, advertisements, and editorial cartoons provide valuable insight into the lives of society. Voices, or narratives, are a huge part of how culture is created and maintained. In healthcare, patients can feel like their voices are not heard. In an attempt to bridge the gap between medical and humanities research and to gain insight into doctor-patient interactions, this analysis asks what ideologies and beliefs are present in medical contexts and how are they represented within the editorial cartoon. Recent studies suggest that mass media as societal discourse may frame or position participants within a society. In this theory of framing, culture is formed from discourse through a reflexive process. Using Kress and Van Leeuwen's research on meaning making, this study will perform a discursive analysis on medical-themed editorial cartoons from *Carpe Diem*, *Rhymes with Orange*, *The Lockhorns,* to *Bizarro.* Through this close reading, explicit and implicit cultural beliefs held about medicine, including practitioners and patients, have been revealed, including the portrayal of the doctor's power over the patient and patient distrust in doctors. Taking into consideration media theory and the analysis of the comics, medical associations and practices may find valuable insight from the opinions and beliefs of not just the authors of these comics but society as a whole, which may prove important as debates over healthcare are ongoing.

Keywords: discursive analysis, comics, graphic medicine, visual semiotics, medical discourse

1. Introduction

With medical and pharmaceutical costs rising and the politicization of healthcare, not a week goes by without mention of the industry in news reporting. New media aside, the print news has been a stronghold news source for centuries covering a wide range of topics. Though journalism is meant to be impartial to cultural values, news-content, including the editorial cartoon, can be filled with the implicit opinions of the author no matter the topic of the story or the medium used. The author's voices and opinions are at the forefront of mass media with potential to influence the masses. These voices are what define and maintain culture. On trend with current debates surrounding healthcare, the analysis presented in this work asks what beliefs are present in medical interactions, how they are represented in mass media such as through editorial cartoons, and the implications that these beliefs have on society. This work uses a methodology that attempts to further relations between medical and humanities scholarship [1, 2].

2. Media and society

It was formerly assumed that mass media had a grand influence on the minds of its viewers with the ability to directly influence their actions [3]. Though recent theorists suggest that media plays a lesser role—rather than directly influencing people's decision-making and actions, societal discourse may frame or position receivers versus producers, or in other words, it may build society by elevating certain roles [1]. In this theory, culture may be viewed as formed from discourse through a reflexive process.

Cultural discourse, such as news media, simultaneously influences and is influenced by culture [4] and may cause the social environment of the individual to slightly change. This could influence cognitive processing in individuals during opinion formation [3]. This theory of framing within cultural discourse follows suit with media communication models of cultivation and media ecology theory. Cultivation theory states that media may cultivate beliefs in viewers [5], while Moreno and Koff's media ecology theory [6] posits that media is within every aspect of society, influences perceptions, and has an inescapable presence. Regardless of the depth of media's grasp in society, it is known to have an influence.

3. From articles to comics

Mass media's influence extends from television commercials, to podcasts, to editorial cartoons; how society feels about various issues is extended into various media. Coming from news-media, the editorial cartoon can be seen as a product of society [7]. Not only do editorial cartoons reflect the artists' opinion on politics and pop culture, but they also reflect, describe, poke fun of, and document the experiences of the everyday person. Just as editorial cartoons are a product of society, they are also a product of their time; ideas and storylines represented reflect cultural beliefs. This extends to the experiences people have with healthcare. Unlike written language contained in articles, comics provide readers with a different way of understanding, coping with complex issues, and creating a deeper bond with the stories told and the information given [1, 8].

One way to further understand the ideologies and beliefs behind comics is to perform a close reading through a discursive framework. In the study of discourse, more than just language is considered—the study of discourse goes well beyond the sentence, including conversations, literature, storytelling, and written, spoken, and visual texts [1]. Through the examination of visual discourses, such as comics, the reader can interpret the way in which the author of the work positions characters within the visual text. These visual texts oftentimes point to the world views of the authors [4, 9].

In an attempt to further understand the view of the creators of a discourse, this analysis employs a visual semiotic framework. Within semiotics, the authors employ on the existence of the study of the sign and the meaning-making practices [10–12].

Meaning-making is the design apparatus combining all elements both visual and textual as well as their size, color, distance, and arrangement. This interplay of design elements simultaneously creating meaning, or perhaps more properly worded, as telling a story, are what the viewer of a discourse interprets as according to Kress and Van Leeuwen's ongoing research and writings [2, 10, 11]. The interpretation may vary depending on the complexity and obviousness of the symbols, signs, and everything else represented. In the meaning-making process, viewers may interpret overt meanings through obvious symbols but also may interpret, subconsciously that is, the covert meanings, or stories, and a visual discourse displays [12].

Using this type of spatial display, art has the power to create deeper imagery and bond with the audience [1]. It is through the analysis of these elements that viewers will discover cultural values and beliefs influencing the visual text [7].

Language or narrative, as created by the ego, works to maintain and construct culture and is the lingua franca of human life. Medicine is to treat the human as a whole and as the body exists within a specific cultural narrative, the discourses of the culture in which the patient exists must be kept in mind. This means not treating the human body as simply a corpse on a cadaver cart, but resisting the medical gaze [13] and treating both the body and the ego [14]. The ego as lived through narrative is one of the few things that set humans apart from other flora and fauna. Whether it is dialogue between a patient and a practitioner, survivor stories, billing statements from an insurance company, or comics depicting medical contexts, language is hugely important in the treatment and cure of the human body.

4. Comics and graphic medicine

Graphic medicine, or comics depicting illness and medical narrative, is a form of storytelling in clinical settings through the use of paneled visual and text. These stories are not limited to that of the patient but can include the family's and practitioner's perspective as well [15]. The study and creation of graphic medicine was born out of a push toward the intersection of the humanities with the medical sciences as a medium with potential to lead clinicians toward a more empathetic approach to medical treatment [8]. Comics in medical contexts can help patients and families come to terms with hospital visits, illness, and trauma.

Aside from graphic medicine created in hospitals, comics with medical contexts, such as popular comics in newspapers, may be viewed as having a similar effect: an ability to create further understanding of difficult topics. This further understanding is partially created through the medium of pen and paper. Drawings are ineffable: they can speak to the human mind in different ways than language and can express things that language cannot. Comics have an accessible and informal approach to the presentation of their information—neither language nor image needs to be intricate to depict intricate meanings. Along with an informal approach, comics often remove the jargonous vocabulary of doctors and replace it with images that are compelling, easier to understand, and create a larger impact on the viewer [15–18].

The comics presented in graphic medicine are "also potentially far more complex, in that a narrative arc provides a scaffold within which an almost endless array of cultural values and preconceptions can be set up, questioned, reinforced, or negotiated" [1, 18]. These comics can present a range of storylines from sweet, to funny, to serious, and to depressing, all of which can appeal to a wide variety of audiences, and are potentially filled with cultural markers [19, 20].

5. Discourse and medical practice

For years, detached concern was an accepted approach to take in the medical field. Detached concern is a method in which doctors may be viewed as looking beyond the patient's narrative and not considering aspects of identity when making diagnoses. In other words, detached concern is an ideology stating that physicians should not engage emotionally with, or be influenced emotionally by, patients [21]. Though envisioned with good intent, this method has been found to be dehumanizing and could be viewed as an aloofness on the job or a lack of caring from the patient's perspective which could further patient distrust [14]. Detached concern stems from the argument that an over-emotional physician's judgment would be clouded and therefore leaving them unable to make the best decisions for their patient. It could also be viewed as a method of burnout prevention for practitioners [16, 22]. Though detached concern is losing favor as an accepted form of practice, it can still be found in the medical field today even as medical care shifts toward developing the patient-practitioner relationship [14].

This idea that attachment, or perhaps viewing the patient with empathy, would negatively affect a physician's ability to diagnose could be interpreted as an extension of the medical gaze. According to Foucault [13], the medical gaze is the concept of separating the patient's ailment and body from their personality and identity, thus allowing the doctor to diagnose without regard to the patient's self. This medical gaze has been criticized as presenting the doctor fully as the decision-maker, or "the eye that knows and decides, the eye that governs" [13]. The mindset of the doctor being in total power could be interpreted as hegemonically positioning patients as the lesser individual in the interaction. This could be viewed as problematic when it comes to treating patients across a variety of cultures. For example, without considering the patient's identity, a doctor may perform a treatment deemed unacceptable or taboo in the culture of the patient; by listening to the patient's story, regardless of lack of medical knowledge, the practitioner could gain valuable insight into the patient's narrative, increase treatment efficacy, and decrease feelings of inferiority within the patient.

By interacting with the patient's narrative, the doctor becomes more invested in the relationship increasing treatment efficacy and patient satisfaction [23]. A big part of the patient's story that could be viewed through graphic medicine is the reclamation of the story that may have been diminished or dehumanized by long hospital visits or indifferent doctors [24]. Spending time in medical institutions can be frustrating, and patients' voices can be replaced by numbers, medical records, and diagnoses [24, 25]. The reclamation or retelling of the patient's story can be a therapeutic process in which the story-teller gets in touch with their own feelings and gets back on track to healthy recovery [26]. By reading graphic medicine, viewers can discover new ways of thinking about hospital visits and illness in order to gain an increased understanding of the patient experience [27, 28].

It is no surprise that in clinical settings, patients may feel powerless. This could be attributed to the all-seeing eye or the medical gaze of the doctor; the powerful apparatus is the doctor possesses that allowing them to diagnose, operate, and drastically change the patient's life without much input from the patient themselves [13]. In some cases, perceived unprofessionalism or insensitivity can cause environments where patients are not speaking up to get the care they need [29]. The professional-looking white laboratory coats were not always the status quo in the medical profession. They could have been adopted to visually distinguish the doctor over others within a medical setting. The white may represent purity or the doctor's vow to do no harm, and the coat itself positions doctors as scientists. Altogether, the outfit could be viewed as positioning physicians as authority figures with the hanging of medical school diplomas as the final mark of authority [30].

When it comes to trusting practitioners, patients are often stressed, vulnerable, and may grant more discretionary power to doctors than normal [31]. Trust is at the forefront of patient care. Without trust in a doctor, a patient may not reveal the full extent of what they are experiencing, and it may prevent proper care. With a disproportionate power dynamic between doctors and patients, as well as the stressful setting of these interactions, it is no surprise that a lack of trust can be found within these interactions. However, trust is of huge importance and may go so far as to positively influence patient outcomes including enhancing the prescribed treatment [31]. Along with enhancing treatment by psychologically building trust, humor is known to play an important role in coping [32]. Humor can help patients come to terms with the psychological trauma that may be experienced in clinical settings.

Though it is not known if the authors of the following comics create specifically from their own illness experiences, these experiences can be viewed as originating from somewhere. Human thought is so nebulously intertwined with society that it would be nearly impossible for authors to eschew cultural context. With the importance of communication in medical contexts and the knowledge of graphic medicine as laden with cultural markers, medical comics have great potential to shed light into the life of the clinical experience.

It is with all this in mind that this study seeks a further understanding of comics and their role in the expression of the human experience in medicine. A random survey of popular cartoons from well-circulated publications was analyzed. The comics surveyed include *Bizarro* by Dan Piraro, *Carpe Diem* by Niklas Eriksson, *Dustin* by Steve Kelley and Jeff Parker, *Intelligent Life* by David Reddick, *Sherman's Lagoon* by Jim Toomey, *The Lockhorns* by Bunny Hoest and John Reiner, *Rhymes with Orange* by Hilary Price, and *Six Chix* by Bannerman et al. [33].

6. Critical comical analysis

Using Kress and Van Leeuwen's research on meaning-making [34], this study will focus on the three metafunctions: the representational, interpersonal, and compositional. The three metafunctions are resources that can be interpreted to find the meaning of a visual [35]. The representational metafunction encompasses all of the things represented in the images, including characters and non-human elements also known as represented participants (RPs) [1]. Usually connected by vectors, or strong lines, the participants within the image tell a story through hand gestures, gazes, and planes [34, 36].

The interpersonal metafunction focuses on how the creators convey meaning to their audiences through the elements of the representational. Various devices can be used by creators of images to connect with their viewers, including demand and social distance. Demand is the use of a character in an image to connect directly with a viewer by appearing to look directly at them [34]. The distance between two characters or elements take from each other can also inform the audience. Characters closer to each other or to the audience are building relationships, while characters further from each other or the audience are not [34].

Where the representational and interpersonal are somewhat sequestered from each other, the compositional examines elements together for effectiveness. Authors have the ability to use salience, or size and focus, iconic displays of emotion, including happiness, anger, and sadness to portray complex emotional situations. The compositional metafunction also looks at modality or whether or not the images are convincing in general [1]. This analysis gains inspiration from the related works of Kaplan-Weinger [34], Juricevic and Horvath [36], Kowalewski [37], and Dalbeto and Oliveira [38], to name a few. This research uses methods founded in the humanities to seek insight into the medical industry and the surrounding ideologies, as well as how these ideologies are conveyed in graphic narrative. The following chart based on Kress and Van Leeuwen's [12] work on metafunctions, with inspiration from the previously cited visual analyses, will serve as the foundation for this study:

I. *Representational metafunction:* In the representational metafunction, who and what is being represented will be considered. Vectors and themes will be gathered from both human and non-human RPs.

II. *Interpersonal metafunction:* This metafunction will examine the interpersonal relationships created between the viewer and author by the use of visual demand and conceptions of social distance.

III. *Compositional metafunction:* This metafunction examines the piece as a whole considering the salience of the RPs and the information they provide, as well as modality and iconic displays of emotion.

With the consideration of the three metafunctions, the selected comics were analyzed in three rounds. During the first round of analysis, the representational metafunctions were considered. The represented participants, both human and non-human, were identified, vectors were highlighted and analyzed, and themes were interpreted. After the representational metafunctions of the comics were mapped out, the interpersonal metafunctions were studied. During this time, the represented participants were examined in relation to the viewer of the comics—the interpersonal relationship between the RP (or the represented participant) and the reader as created through social distance and visual demand was identified and analyzed. Finally, the compositional metafunctions were examined. The comics as a whole were studied to determine which RPs were most salient; facial displays of emotion were interpreted, and modality was considered.

For each of the metafunctions belonging to each of the comics, the author created a spreadsheet to organize the results side-by-side for a comparison. This comparison yielded the major themes as identified in this study.

About 24 comics were chosen for analysis from King Features Syndicate. As syndicated in around 5000 newspapers worldwide, the comics of King Features Syndicate have distinguishable breadth, potentially reaching millions of readers. After choosing a syndicate with extensive reach in order to use data that have measurable influence, the data pool was selected. On King Features' website, 24 comics were chosen at random using key words such as *doctor, nurse, medicine,* and *illness*, entered into an appendix, and assigned an arbitrary letter (a–x). To further randomize and refine this selection, an Excel algorithm was used to select four comics from the data pool. Each letter (a–x) was entered in a spreadsheet and assigned a random number. Through the Excel RANDBETWEEN function, each letter was given a number (1–24). The final step of the selection process used the Filter and Sort function to order the numbers (and the letters) from lowest to largest (between 1 and 24). The four lowest numbers were selected for a more thorough investigation as presented below.

7. Summary of findings

After a close reading of the four comics selected, the following themes have been identified: (a) the salience of the doctor over the patient, (b) the expression of vectors, (c) the salience of white coats and hanging diplomas, (d) patient distrust of medical professionals, (e) humor, and (f) the role of women in medical care. To merit analysis, discussed themes occurred at least twice within the comics analyzed.

a. Salience of the doctor over the patient

In many of the comics surveyed, the doctors were often portrayed in positions more salient than that of the patient. This presents a rather interesting dichotomy between the competing represented participants as those that created these cartoons are likely composing from the patient's perspective and have still chosen, whether consciously or not, to portray the doctor in a position of power over the patient.

b. Vectors from the doctor's gaze

One of the tools used in comics to give meaning, or tell stories, is that of vectors. Vectors are lines that are drawn—whether verbatim lines, or lines creatively displayed—and used to direct the reader's eye in order of importance. Of the comics analyzed, many vectors were drawn from the eye-level plane of the doctor. In many cases, the doctor is portrayed looking down upon the patient or looking through the deep sides of the eyes toward the patient. This could be interpreted as the doctor being portrayed as higher status than patients, or the doctor as being annoyed or unbothered by the patients.

c. Diploma and coat

From a critical perspective, the white laboratory coat and the framed and hanging medical diploma of the doctors can be seen as setting the tone of the interaction. Framing the interaction by positioning the doctor as the one with power as expressed through the coat and diploma could be compared to the scepter and cape of that of royal authority. By extension, without such agency-granting artifacts, the patient may be portrayed as inferior.

d. Patient distrust

Within the selected comics for analysis, many of the authors portray the patients as dumb or air-headed. This paints an interesting perspective as the authors likely have more experience from the side of the patient than that of the practitioner. Through the portrayal of patients as dumb or air-headed, the authors could be interpreted as expressing feelings of inferiority. These feelings of inferiority, as displayed through visual and textual evidence, may lead to distrust in the exam room and are supported through both visual and textual evidence. Doctors are often portrayed as aloof or even lazy when it comes to practitioner-patient interactions, which could be viewed as adding to patient misgivings. Nurses, however, are sometimes portrayed as compensating for these incoherencies by extending compassion to the patient, which the doctor does not.

e. Funny, Doc

Comics are known and often assumed to be humorous [39]. Some of the comics analyzed give way to humor. Though, perhaps these comics, while using humorous appeals, are actually showing readers something further. Humor is a known coping mechanism for many when experiencing increased stress levels during medical visits. These comics could be seen as appealing to humor as a means to make due with tough situations. That humor used in this way could suggest that medical experiences are stressful in and of themselves.

f. Women can be doctors too

Within this data pool, all doctors are portrayed as male. Though fewer instances of the portrayal of nurses occur, when nurses are depicted, they always appear as female. The viewer may interpret an implicit bias toward men in the role as physicians, though recent statistics show that the number of women enrolling in medical school is higher than men [40].

8. Meet the comics!

8.1 *Bizarro* by Wayno and Dan Piraro

Bizzaro is a highly satirical comic with larger than life characters and a bizarre worldview. Starting in 1985, this comic has been entertaining readers with explosives and thought-provoking dry humor. The author offers eccentric visualizations and commentaries on the oddities of our everyday life and culture; oftentimes poking fun of things, we may consider normal. To make commentaries on society and human interaction, the author places visual devices in the comics, including things such as The Eyeball of Observation, The Fish of Humility, and The Crown of Power to name a few. This comic has won many awards such as "best newspaper cartoon panel."

In this frame (**Figure 1**) by Wayno and Piraro, the audience is invited to view what appears to be an exam room interaction. The authors use vivid colors which draw attention to the patient and a rather minimalistic style throughout the rest of the image. In this image, the viewer can see the patient sitting atop an exam table and a doctor standing next to them. The doctor is wearing a white laboratory coat with a stethoscope around their neck and a reflex-hammer in hand. The patient is dressed as a clown and above the scene is hanging what appears to be a diploma from a medical school.

In this image, the main represented participants include the doctor, the patient, the exam room, and the diploma. As it appears, the doctor is in the middle of an exam having just tested the patient's gag reflex. In a word bubble, the doctor states, "Your gag reflexes are fine but we still need to get your jinks a little higher." The major themes in this image include the salience of the white coat and diploma, and the portrayal of the patient as of a lesser intellectual level.

8.1.1 Representational

At first glance, the eye of the viewer may go straight to the patient then travel along vectors from the patient's head, to the diploma, to the doctor. While the patient is where the eye seems to land at first glance, this could be viewed as the authors placing emphasis on how doctors may make patients feel belittled. Whether or not the patient is an actual clown or is portrayed as a clown in this image may not matter—clowns are traditionally used to denote people who are not to be taken seriously. For example, one might say about a friend who is perceived as unintelligent that they should go to clown college. Clowns are also often portrayed in media as clumsy, humorous, or dopey. This representation of the patient as a clown could be seen as serving to increase the gap between perceived intellectual levels between the doctor and the patient. The patient is displayed as sitting, as most patients are; sitting is a weaker social position than standing in many circumstances.

8.1.2 Interpersonal

The represented participants within this panel are represented in close social distance to each other; this could be interpreted as suggesting a closer relationship

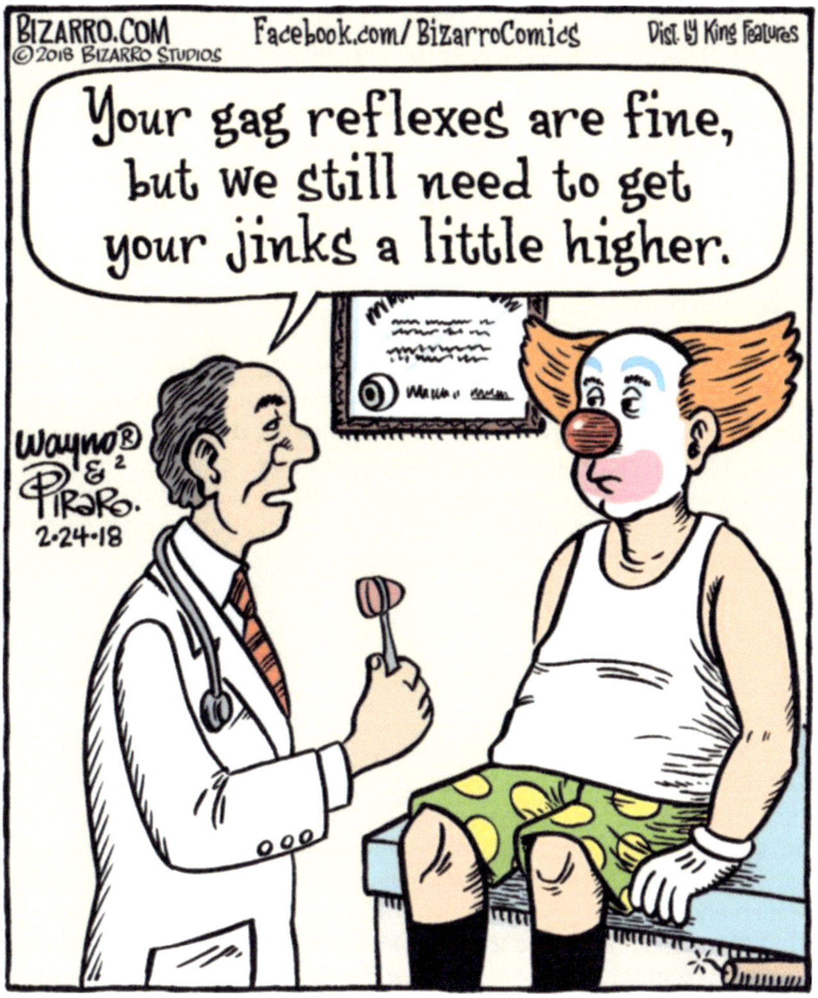

Figure 1.
Bizarro *by Dan Piraro and Wayno, published on February 24, 2018 [41].*

between this doctor and patient even with the anticipated torment that comes with "jinks" testing. Though the two human RPs are close in proximity to one another, neither are directly addressing the reader of the strip. Even as not directly facing the reader, the reader may still interpret the patient's face as an iconic facial expression of anger or perhaps more accurately, frustration. As far as modality goes, this image is purely fictional in its situation, though it may be argued to still have a sense of believability to it. The viewer of this comic might find it obvious that this situation would never happen in a medical setting, but at the same time, they recognize the frustration the authors may be trying to convey.

8.1.3 Compositional

Another important theme is the salience or positioning of the doctor's diploma and laboratory coat. Represented participants in this frame are given the positions of power. The white laboratory coat is a symbol of power. It is known that doctors wear such coats to stand out among colleagues and patients [42]. This practice as is manifest in this comic form could be seen as drawing attention to the prestige associated with medical practice. The diploma could also be interpreted as a symbol of power. The diploma is more salient in this frame than the white coat and is seemingly looming over the room. This framed document could be interpreted as an artifact that lends authority to the practitioner. The diploma also contains an eye peering toward the doctor, directing the reader's attention to them. This could be interpreted as the authors suggesting that the doctor has the power of audience in this interaction. Along with the hidden eyeball, under the exam table is a stick of dynamite. This can be seen as contrasting the eye: stating that while eyes are on the doctor, the patient may find themselves in trouble.

8.1.4 Modality of the metafunctions

This comic by Wayno and Piraro uses the three metafunctions to tell a story that is anything but superficial. At the surface, someone reading the comic might see a funny exam room scene. But with a closer examination, themes of power dichotomies between practitioners and patients are represented. As we know from media and cultural studies, both culture and media are interdependent and constantly shaping one another. Whether or not the authors intentionally represented these themes to publicly disclose their opinions on medical practice, or whether they did so subconsciously, these themes have become present in this comic and are a byproduct of society.

8.2 *Carpe Diem* by Niklas Eriksson

From aliens, to pets, to demons, and to ghosts, you will never know what *Carpe Diem* will hold. Translated as "seize the day," this comic is about a day in the life of a seemingly endless number of characters. Tackling issues such as iPhone versus Android, self-automated cars, and three-dimensional printers, the author offers commentary on contemporary life. Along with the contemporary is the ancient and the metaphorical—from cavemen, to Vikings, and to knights, historical humor can be found. And for figurative scenes, the commentary is no less humorous; it is simply coming from the mouths of fictional characters, such as the Grim Reaper, the Devil, dogs and cats, or even talking volcanos. This satirical panel has a far reach and has received international attention and awards.

In Niklas Eriksson's comic (**Figure 2**), we see the first example as shown in this analysis of a doctor and what is arguably a nurse in the frame alongside the patient with the identifying factor being the nurse's cap. This picture portrays a doctor attempting to read an X-ray and a nurse intervening. This panel uses pastel colors and is simplistic in illustration.

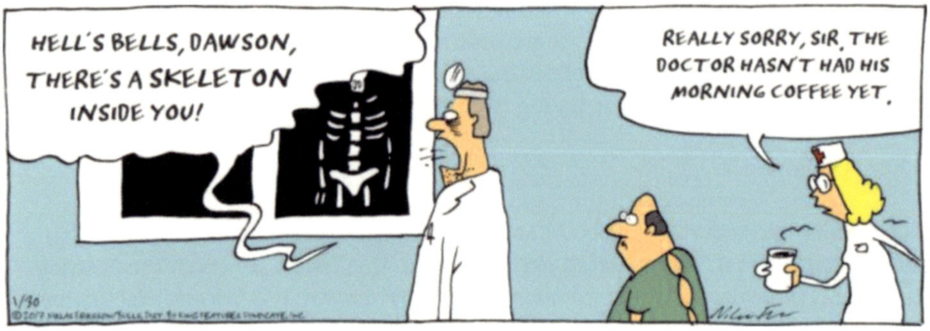

Figure 2.
Carpe Diem *by Niklas Eriksson, published on January 30, 2017 [43].*

The main represented participants in this image include the doctor, the patient, the nurse, and the word-bubbles. In this image, the doctor appears to be yelling at the X-ray atop of the X-ray film viewer and saying, "Hell's bells, Dawson, there's a skeleton inside you!" As the patient looks dumbfounded, a nurse is hurrying behind with a mug of coffee replying, "Really sorry, sir. The doctor hasn't had his morning coffee yet." This panel introduces the patient's distrust of the doctor and the salience of the white coat.

8.2.1 Representational

In this panel, the doctor is arguably portrayed in the strongest position and claims authority through the framing-work done by their laboratory coat. Although the nurse is dressed in a similar white coat, her position of authority is questioned because of nurse's cap which could be viewed as outdated and perhaps insulting that a nurse is portrayed in this particular uniform, and is arguably portrayed as female, may be interpreted as a reflection of society's view of nurses in healthcare.

The patient in this image has the least powerful position as can be reckoned by their lack of height. Even as the doctor is portrayed as aloof, the patient too could be interpreted as being portrayed as rather goofy, dumbfounded, or inferior to the doctor who is calling the shots, no matter how off they may be. By illustrating the patient with such a mountainous head and bulbous nose, the author could be viewed as suggesting the patient's inferiority through humorous assets.

8.2.2 Interpersonal

With a closer social distance, the author of this comic may be suggesting something about the relationship between the three human RPs. Compared with the other comics, the people in this image are portrayed from the waist up suggesting close proximity, which could be viewed as an invitation to gain a closer relationship with the RPs in this panel.

8.2.3 Compositional

Along with this close proximity, the author may be reaching out to the readers by using an iconic representation of anger in the doctor's face. This representation is immediately recognizable, and the reader of this comic may quickly connect with this RP. This image is both believable and unbelievable. It may be interpreted as highly believable that a groggy doctor may make a mistake without caffeine, but could be viewed as implausible that a doctor could have such huge oversight.

The portrayal of the patient also gives insight into their feelings. With bulging eyes and a slightly opened mouth, the patient could be interpreted as dumbfounded at the doctor's incoherence on the job. This portrayal may lend itself to the theme of patients distrust in medical professionals.

8.2.4 Modality of the metafunctions

In Eriksson's work, readers can interpret the author as highlighting the perceived aloofness of doctors, the patient's distrust of practitioners, the authority of doctors as partially maintained by the laboratory coat, and the positioning of doctors versus nurses. Arguably, the most prominent theme in this panel as can be interpreted by the viewer is that of patient distrust and the aloofness of medical professionals. The author of this comic uses coffee-humor and alludes to the doctor's lack of caffeine as the source of incoherence. As the reader may interpret, even without coffee, a doctor should not be so much aloof as to misread an X-ray in this way. The patient's bulging eyes give away their emotion as they stand behind the doctor.

8.3 *The Lockhorns* by Bunny Hoest and John Reiner

To make fun of married couples and the trials and tribulations they experience, the author illustrates sticky scenarios through two recurring characters: Loretta and Leroy Lockhorn. Whether it is Leroy rolling eyes after Loretta says something, or Loretta telling the therapist how Leroy never helps around the house, readers cannot help but relate to this couple's experiences. Leroy is a stark contrast to Loretta with a strong personality, stubbornness, and ability to sit for hours in front of a TV sleeping. When not worried about Leroy, Loretta is a shopping addict and spends more than any person should. Loretta loves to cook and helps Leroy's strong character type.

In this image (**Figure 3**) by Hoest and Reiner, readers view the inside of an exam room in a doctor's office. In the upper right, a doctor is portrayed holding an X-ray, and in the off-center left, the patient sitting on an exam table. The color choices of the authors are very minimal with two tones of a yellowish-beige being the most vivid. The scene of the exam room is represented with straight lines and angles and is altogether very uncluttered. The patient is wearing socks and a hospital gown and the doctor is wearing a laboratory coat.

The main represented participants in this frame include the patient, the doctor, the diploma, the laboratory coat, the X-ray, and the exam room. The patient as a represented participant in this frame is portrayed wearing a blue hospital gown, sitting down on an exam table, and looking sideways toward the doctor, and appears to be irate. The doctor as an RP in this image is portrayed facing away from and glancing at the patient from the side, wearing a laboratory coat, and holding an X-ray of what could be interpreted as a knee joint, and appears to be mid-sentence. The exam room as a whole is represented in a minimalistic or sterile way with one of the focal points being the framed med-school diploma. In terms of the lack of

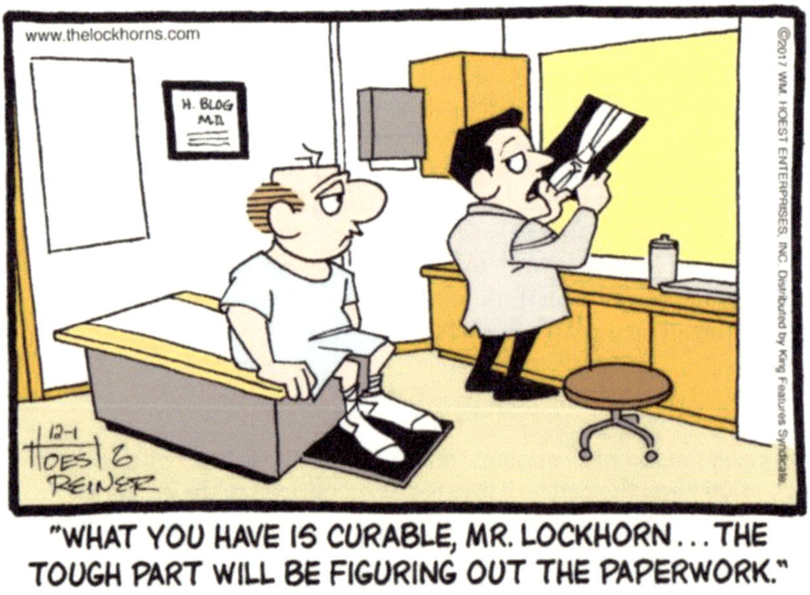
www.thelockhorns.com
H. BLOG M.D.
©2017 WM. HOEST ENTERPRISES, INC. Distributed by King Features Syndicate.
12-1 HOEST & REINER
"WHAT YOU HAVE IS CURABLE, MR. LOCKHORN... THE TOUGH PART WILL BE FIGURING OUT THE PAPERWORK."

Figure 3.
The Lockhorns *by Bunny Hoest and John Reiner, published on December 1, 2017 [44].*

detail, or sterility of the scene, the authors could be portraying a sense of bleakness or an emotionally cold experience in a medical context. At the bottom of the frame, the doctor is saying to the patient, "What you have is curable, Mr. Lockhorn...the tough part will be figuring out the paperwork." The themes identified in this frame include the salience of the diploma and the coat, vectors from the doctor's gaze, and patient distrust.

8.3.1 Representational

In this image, the medical school diploma seems to dominate the horizontal plane. Framed with thick black lines and surrounded by empty white space, the eye tends to wander to the diploma. In this image, the laboratory coat is neither as salient as the diploma nor as salient in comparison with the other comics. In fact, the laboratory coat could be interpreted as grey in this image. While the diploma could be seen as hovering over the room as with the previous example, vectors are a stronger form at play within this image.

Looking over their shoulder and down the patient, the doctor could be interpreted as positioned or framed in a position of power via vectors. Not only standing is a more powerful position than sitting, the position in the upper right-hand corner places the doctor at a higher eye-level-plane than the patient. The reader might question why the authors have decided to portray the doctor speaking to the patient in this way while giving a diagnosis or speaking of a cure rather than turning around and addressing the patient directly. This could be interpreted as the doctor placing a higher-level importance on handling the X-ray and other tasks than the patient's needs for an empathetic delivery of medical information.

8.3.2 Interpersonal

The two human RPs in this image are not portrayed in close proximity—this far distance between them suggests a degree of separation. While the doctor and patient are looking at each other, neither is creating visual demand with the audience of this image. However, through the iconic display of anger on the patient's face, the reader is invited to empathize with the RP. Along with the distance between the two human RPs, the authors have chosen to show the reader the entire bodies of these characters; by doing so, the authors have presented the scene as further away, or perhaps given us the perspective of an outsider looking in, rather than being up close and a part of the conversation.

8.3.3 Compositional

Through the facial expression of the patient in response to the doctor's comments, the reader may interpret the distrust of or frustration with medical care by the patient. The eyes of the patient may be viewed as frustrated or defeated upon the delivery of this news while already out of their comfort zone from being in the hospital. This may be viewed as a metacommentary on societal opinions of medical care in the United States and that of the authors, however, infinitely intertwined the two may be.

8.3.4 Modality of the metafunctions

Discursive analysis of this comic by Hoest and Reiner yields themes of patient distrust or dissatisfaction, positioning of the doctor at a higher level, and the authority of the medical-school diploma. While looking at this image in terms of modality scope, considering all of the elements, the reader may interpret this image as highly plausible and likely to have happened.

8.4 *Rhymes with Orange* by Hilary Price

With over 400 non-recurring characters, the author still has not found anything that rhymes with orange. This high energy comic strip examines the universal truths of the ordinary: in-laws, driving, pets, children, and love. With recreations of daily life of its readers, this comic often points out just how weird, yet wonderful, humanity is.

In this comic titled *Modern Medicine* (**Figure 4**) by Hillary Price, readers are taken into a care unit. This comic has livelier colors than the previous with pastels of green, orange, and blue. The author pays little attention to extraneous detail with a focus on the image at whole. In the first frame of the comic, the title of this strip is introduced. At the bottom of the panel, the reader can see the doctor asking the patient "Can you give me a hand?" In the second panel, the reader of this comic gets a zoomed-out image of the scene. A doctor is in an exam room looking for their stethoscope which is apparently tangled up with headphones. The patient is sitting in their bed watching as the doctor says, "Shoot, my earbuds."

The main represented participants in these two panels include the doctor, the white coat, the patient, the earbud-stethoscope knot, and the patient's room. The doctor in these two panels is portrayed wearing a white coat with business attire underneath. The patient is portrayed as presumably elderly, with grey hair, and glasses. The room is portrayed rather bare, lending attention to the other RPs. Themes contained within these panels include the aloofness of the doctor, the salience of the laboratory coat, and humor.

8.4.1 Representational

Surrounded by a sea of green, the doctor's laboratory coat seems to stick out as a prominent represented participant within this image. Combining the length of the two panels together, the doctor and their coat are in the true center of the comic. The center position lends power to this RP.

Another theme that can be seen across the data pool of comics, including this panel specifically, is the perceived or illustrated aloofness of doctors. As the reader follows the composition of the art, their eye moves from the foot of the bed up to the patient's face who is looking at the knot. From vectors drawn, emphasis is placed on the knot that the stethoscope and earbuds are in. This knot could be interpreted as a symbol for the doctor's mind while making rounds. Perhaps the author has been

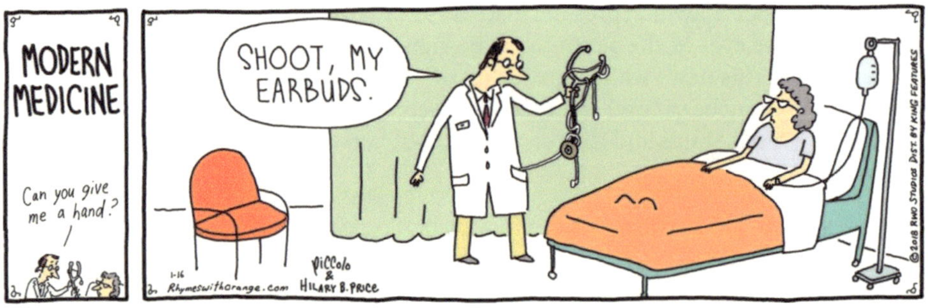

Figure 4.
Rhymes with Orange *by Hilary Price, published on January 16, 2018 [45].*

a patient and felt, consciously or subconsciously, that doctors can be distracted by out-of-hospital issues. Along with distracted doctors comes distrust in healthcare and healthcare professionals. For example, if a patient was in pre-op and a doctor was seemingly distracted or not fully present, the patient could suffer higher levels of distress.

8.4.2 Interpersonal

The fact that the author has chosen to portray the doctor and the patient at a further social distance may suggest something toward the relationship between these two RPs. In the same way, the author has not utilized any form of directly addressing the reader of this comic to enhance viewing. However, with the analysis of facial expressions, the reader may get a strong sense of the situation. While not necessarily iconic displays of emotion through facial features, the reader could envision themselves as the patient or the doctor and imagine themselves in this context. This image has both believable and unbelievable aspects to it: that a doctor would keep a stethoscope in their pocket with earbuds rather than taking a different approach to avoid such tangled circumstances could be viewed as fiction; however, readers may look into this setting and empathize with how easy it can be to get earbuds tangled in a knot.

8.4.3 Compositional

These two comics have a sense of humor interjected into their illustration. The way the author portrays the expression on the doctor's face versus the expression on the patient's face could be interpreted as using humor in stressful situations to cope, or perhaps to relate to those who have felt in similar ways.

8.4.4 Modality of the metafunctions

This comic by price portraying a doctor entering a patient's room continues the trend of media portraying—or reflecting—societal distrust of practitioners, the use of white coats to position practitioners over patients, and humor as used in stressful situations.

9. Discussion and conclusions

Through this close reading *of Carpe Diem, Rhymes with Orange, The Lockhorns,* and *Bizarro*, explicit and implicit cultural beliefs held about medicine, including practitioners and patients, have been revealed through the study of signs and symbols and the meaning-making work they perform [10, 11]. It could be argued that these beliefs as conveyed through comics are more salient than those in the articles of the same newspapers as comics provide readers more tools for understanding than words do on their own [1, 34].

For example, the authors of the comics usually portrayed doctors in positions of higher power. As we know from Kress and Van Leeuwen [12] and de Rothewelle [1], and through the findings of Kaplan-Weinger's study of graphic medicine [34], the placement of a represented participant and the distance between represented participants within an image are meaningful. Through these four comics, the doctors were portrayed in positions of higher power. For example, just as Kaplan-Weinger analyzed the planes of characters represented in comics, it could be viewed that the doctors are portrayed on higher planes than patients and looking down upon them when addressing the patients. These vectors painted with the eyes of doctors and patients serve as valuable insight. Also lending emphasis to the doctors in these comics are the artifacts that give them agency and power. Kress and Van Leeuwen [12] demonstrate that the salience of an object within an image is a meaning-making function used by authors. Kowalewski found that signs representing cultural ideologies created to lend a form of cognitive salience in the readership have impact [37]. In the same way, representations of medical school diplomas and white laboratory coats could be portrayed as signs or icons representing implicit cultural values and usually positioned in more salient forms than that of other RPs. These visual artifacts could be interpreted as visually separating doctors from nurses and patients within these comics. These two items serve as tangible artifacts that appear to lend power to the doctor's position.

Whereas the diploma and the laboratory coat lend power to the doctor's position, within this data set and the four comics on which the close reading was performed, the position of doctor or physician is always portrayed as a male-presenting role. According to Schiffrin [9] and Davies and Harré [4], identity is performed and co-constructed through positioning. By positioning doctors as above those who they treat, the authors may be reinforcing the idea of a doctor's autonomy. Kress and Van Leeuwen [12] also posit that proximity in relation to other humans can be used to interpret meaning. As is known from similar studies, such as that of Kaplan-Weinger [34], the closer two human RPs are portrayed to each other, the more likely they may be to become intimate, which is typically represented by a friendly conversation or a handshake. On the other hand, characters portrayed further from each other could be interpreted as seeking no interaction. In the comics, the doctors were usually portrayed in a distant proximity to the patient, which could be interpreted as a lack of interest by the doctor in becoming too close to the patient.

The analysis of these four comics in particular shows that they all portray patients as inferior to doctors. This could be viewed as an extension of a patient's distrust of doctors and a visual representation of how patients may be made to feel during interactions with doctors. Along with this distrust of doctors is what could be viewed as the portrayal of doctors acting aloof or pre-occupied at times when they could be more attentive to patients. These portrayals could be viewed as made through vectors and continued through the compositional metafunctions [2], including the use of written language. These portrayals of the doctors' and patients' opinions of each other could also be interpreted through facial features. The idea of patient's distrust of doctors is more of a metaphorical device painted by the visual text such as the ones Juricevic and Horvath found in their work. Whereas metaphors may not have a specific and previously defined sign and signified correlation, icons do [36]. Anger, sadness, and happiness are all posited to be iconic emotional displays, that is, whenever these faces are made, one immediately knows what the other is feeling [1]. This window to the feelings of the represented participants lends ease to the reader when empathizing with the portrayed characters.

A lesser theme in the four comics examined in this analysis is the lack of portrayal of female presenting doctors. The author pays no homage to a binary gender system, though realizes these comics were created in a society where such a system is upheld by the cultural majority. Just as Dalbeto and Oliveira [38] located cultural stereotypes of women of color through visual analysis, this study found stereotypes of women in medical practice; within the male and female stereotypes as represented in these comics, doctors are always portrayed by men, and nurses are always portrayed by women. In the four closely dissected comics, and throughout the entire data pool of 24 comics, the results remain the same. Humor is another less prominent theme as displayed throughout the comics and is trickier to grasp as the medium itself is traditionally considered to be humorous. However, these comics could be interpreted as containing humor to cope with stressful situations during medical exams and hospital stays. For example, in *Carpe Diem*, it is humorous that the doctor has misidentified the X-ray, but it is also a scary situation as one wrong move in a procedure could be life-threatening. Perhaps it is the author's way of attempting to distress a portrayal of a situation, where a doctor is aloof on the job.

These comics are products of the society, and they were created in and may be found to reflect the ideologies of that society [7]. Cohn et al. [46] have found that the interpretation of visuals and rhetorical devices in comics is culturally dependent. Whereas all of the identified themes and ideologies presented in this analysis may yield great insight into the medical industry, they may not be the representative of the various cultures of the world. For example, the push toward a relationship-based approach to the doctor-patient relationship may be a product of United States culture and may not transfer over—the person reading these comics as distributed in India may not elicit the same responses. Just as we know that comics can help bridge the understanding of difficult topics and create a response in the readership [8], it is also known that if comics do a poor job at depicting their story, the reader can become all the more confused as Farinella points out [47].

As Grice [48] states, all communication must uphold four maxims to be effective: the maxims of quantity, quality, relevance, and manner. Viewing these comics outside of their original cultural context could be viewed as violating communicative maxims and would almost certainly be cause for different results. For example, in terms of the iconography of the white laboratory coat and the framed medical school diploma, the maxim of relevance might be violated in a culture that does not practice Western medicine. In other cultures, a doctor or a healer might be designated with a different type of attire and retained different types of artifacts on display to assert their knowledge.

Another consideration for these comics is the reflexive nexus that continues to construct culture by creators and receivers of discourse [4]. These comics have the potential to provide insight in what may be viewed in a positive light by creating change and improvement in medical care—or these comics may create a spiral effect that continues to sway popular opinion of medicine. For example, news media coverage of certain events is known to create an illusory truth effect [49]. This portrayal of what could be interpreted as negative ideologies surrounding medical care could continue to foster negative ideologies when medical associations and practitioners are moving in a different direction.

Whereas these comics may be a representation of the author's beliefs and a reflection of cultural beliefs in general, just as Dalbeto and Oliviera have found [38], these comics are in distributed newspapers worldwide and may have a sizable impact. After all, comics are a product of the culture they are created in, and the artistic choices of the authors offer valuable cultural insight and potential to influence readers [38]. It is no longer assumed that the media has such an intrusive influence on the life of the individual; it is suggested that this discourse may aid in the framing of represented participants [1, 3]. With the reflexive nature of media in mind, the co-construction of cultural discourses by authors and audiences [4], these media may be viewed as a reflection of cultural opinion and having the ability to influence cultural opinion [3].

Taking into consideration media theory and the analysis of the comics, medical associations and practices may find valuable insight into the opinions and beliefs of not just the authors of these comics but of society as a whole. According to Dalbeto and Oliveira [38], "a critical analysis of comics, and of any cultural asset, is necessary because [...] they are not free of ideologies." With this in mind, the themes of doctors as more powerful and more important than patients, doctors presenting as one of the two culturally accepted genders rather than the other, aloofness of doctors on the job, and distrust in doctors and the medical system were interpreted. These themes could be interpreted largely as the reflections of societal opinions of medical practice and could be taken as pointers to improve patient satisfaction by reducing stress through building doctor-patient trust [5, 6]. Comics pull readers in and help them to imagine themselves in the situations pictured; therefore, practitioners may find comics as a powerful tool for improving patient care and understanding the patient's experience [34].

10. Limitations and future research

This research purposely works with a small sample size from one news syndication to make data manageable. To establish a farther-reaching analysis of how medicine is represented in editorial cartoons and the influence these cartoons have on culture, a larger sample size from multiple sources could broaden the results. To facilitate a scope this large, a data-analytic technology to aid research would be necessary. Along with a larger scope, it is known that images may mean different things in different cultures and thus would be worthy of dissection from a cross-cultural standpoint [46].

Acknowledgements

This work was made possible with the advice of my colleagues at Harry S. Truman College and Northeastern Illinois University. Permissions granted by King Features Syndicate. Thanks to those who helped copy edit.

Author details

Jonathan Comyn de Rothewelle
The Department of Communication and The Reading Center, Harry S. Truman College, Chicago, United States

*Address all correspondence to: jcomynderothewelle@gmail.com

References

[1] de Rothewelle JC. Comics and medical narrative: A visual semiotic dissection of graphic medicine. Journal of Graphic Novels and Comics [Internet]. 2018 Oct:1-27. DOI: 10.1080/21504857.2018.1530271

[2] Kress G, Van Leeuwen T. Multimodal Discourse: The Modes and Media of Contemporary Communication. Oxford, UK: Oxford University Press; 2001

[3] Borah P. Media Effects Theory. The International Encyclopedia of Political Communication [Internet]. Hoboken, New Jersey: John Wiley & Sons, Inc.; 2016 Jan. pp. 1-12. DOI: 10.1002/9781118541555.wbiepc156

[4] Davies B, Harre R. Positioning: The discursive production of selves. Journal for the Theory of Social Behaviour [Internet]. 1990 Mar;**20**(1):43-63. DOI: 10.1111/j.1468-5914.1990.tb00174.x

[5] Gerbner G, Gross L, Morgan M, Signorielli N, Shahnahan J. Growing up with television: Cultivation process. In: Bryant J, Zillmann G, editors. Media Effects: Advances in Theory and Research. Mahwah, NJ: Erlbaum; 2002. pp. 43-67

[6] Moreno MA, Koff R. 11. Media theories and the facebook influence model. In: The Psychology of Social Networking [Internet]. Vol. 1. De Gruyter Open; 2015 Jan. DOI: 10.1515/9783110473780-01

[7] Brienza C. Producing comics culture: a sociological approach to the study of comics. Journal of Graphic Novels & Comics [Internet]. 2010 Dec;**1**(2):105-119. DOI: 10.1080/21504857.2010.528638

[8] Williams ICM. Graphic medicine: comics as medical narrative. Medical Humanities [Internet]. 2012 Jan;**38**(1):21-27. DOI: 10.1136/medhum-2011-010093

[9] Schiffrin D. Approaches to discourse. Blackwell Textbooks in Linguistics. Oxford: Blackwell; 1994

[10] Kress G. Multimodality: Challenges to thinking about language. TESOL Quarterly [Internet]. 2000;**34**(2):337. DOI: 10.2307/3587959

[11] Thibault PJ. Editorial: Social semiotics. In: The Semiotic Review of Books. Vol. 4. Ontario, Canada: University of Toronto Press; 1993. p. 1

[12] Kress G, Van Leeuwen T. Reading Images. Routledge; 2006 Mar. DOI: 10.4324/9780203619728

[13] Foucault M. The Birth of the Clinic. Routledge; 2002 Nov. DOI: 10.4324/9780203406373

[14] Halpern J. What is clinical empathy? Journal of General Internal Medicine [Internet]. 2003 Aug;**18**(8):670-674. DOI: 10.1046/j.1525-1497.2003.21017.x

[15] Green MJ. Graphic storytelling and medical narrative: The use of comics in medical education. In: The Graphic Medicine Manifesto. University Park, Pennsylvania: The Pennsylvania State University Press; 2015

[16] Czerwiec MK. Taking Turns: Stories from HIV/AIDS Care Unit 371. University Park, Pennsylvania: The Pennsylvania State University Press; 2017

[17] Chute H. Comics as literature? Reading graphic narrative. PMLA [Internet]. 2008 Mar;**123**(2):452-465. DOI: 10.1632/pmla.2008.123.2.452

[18] Bateman JA. Text and Image. Abingdon, United Kingdom: Routledge; 2014 May. DOI: 10.4324/9781315773971

[19] Smith ST. Who gets to speak? The making of comics scholarship. In: The

Graphic Medicine Manifesto. University Park, Pennsylvania: The Pennsylvania State University Press; 2015

[20] Squier SM. The uses of graphic medicine for engaged scholarship. In: The Graphic Medicine Manifesto. University Park, Pennsylvania: The Pennsylvania State University Press; 2015

[21] Halpern J. From Detached Concern to Empathy. Oxford, UK: Oxford University Press; 2001 Jun. DOI: 10.1093/acprof:osobl/9780195111194.001.0001

[22] Lampert B, Unterrainer C, Seubert CT. Exhausted through client interaction—Detached concern profiles as an emotional resource over time? PLoS One [Internet]. 2019 May;**14**(5):e0216031. DOI: 10.1371/journal.pone.0216031

[23] Laub D, Felman S. Bearing witness or the vicissitudes of listening. In: Testimony: Crises of Witnessing in Literature, Psychoanalysis, and History. New York, London: Routledge; 1992. pp. 57-74

[24] Frank AW. The Wounded Storyteller. Chicago, United States: University of Chicago Press; 1997. DOI: 10.7208/chicago/9780226067360.001.0001

[25] Godfrey, A, Mould, E. But who is this story for?: Representation and responsibility in autobiographical comics [video podcast]. 2014. Available from: http://www.graphicmedicine.org/new-podcast-andrew-godfrey-emma-mould/

[26] Billington J. Is Literature Healthy? Oxford, United Kingdom: Oxford University Press; 2016

[27] Green MJ, Myers KR. Graphic medicine: Use of comics in medical education and patient care. British Medical Journal [Internet]. 2010 Mar;**340**(mar03 2):c863-c863. DOI: 10.1136/bmj.c863

[28] Shwed A. Crisis Averted in Infinite Lives: Utilizing Comics as Clinical Art Therapy. New York, United States: Intima; 2016

[29] Tsuda M. De-stigmatizing Mental Illness through Graphic Medicine. SKMC. Philadelphia, Pennsylvania: Jefferson Digital Commons; 2019

[30] Jones VA. The white coat: Why not follow suit? JAMA [Internet]. 1999 Feb;**281**(5):478. DOI: 10.1001/jama.281.5.478-jms0203-5-1

[31] Goold SD. Trust, distrust and trustworthiness. Journal of General Internal Medicine [Internet]. 2002 Jan;**17**(1):79-81. DOI: 10.1046/j.1525-1497.2002.11132.x

[32] Bellert JL. Humor. Cancer Nursing [Internet]. 1989 Apr;**12**(2):65-70. DOI: 10.1097/00002820-198904000-00002

[33] According to Reed Brennan Media Associates. Available from: https://www.rbma.com/about-us/

[34] Kaplan-Weinger J. Addressing loss and resilience: Informing patient care through comic narratives. Atrium: The Report of the Northwestern Medical Humanities and Bioethics Program. Evanston, Illinois: Northwestern Center for Bioethics; 2012;(10)

[35] Stoian C. Analysing images: A social semiotic perspective. Scientific Bulletin of the Politehnica University of Timisoara Transactions on Modern Languages. 2015;**14**(1):23-30

[36] Juricevic I, Horvath AJ. Analysis of motions in comic book cover art: Using pictorial metaphors. Comics Grid: Journal of Comics Scholarship [Internet]. 2016 Apr;**6**(1). DOI: 10.16995/cg.71

[37] Kowalewski H. Heart is for love: Cognitive salience and visual metonymies in comics. The Comics Grid: Journal of Comics Scholarship [Internet]. 2018;**8**(1). DOI: 10.16995/cg.117

[38] Dalbeto L do C, Oliveira AP. Oh my goddess: Anthropological thoughts on the representation of Marvel's Storm and the Legacy of Black Women in comics. The Comics Grid: Journal of Comics Scholarship [Internet]. 2015 Jun;**4**(1). DOI: 10.5334/cg.bd

[39] Overholser JC. Sense of humor when coping with life stress. Personality and Individual Differences [Internet]. 1992 Jul;**13**(7):799-804. DOI: 10.1016/0191-8869(92)90053-r

[40] Johnson M. The healthcare future is female. Athena insight: Athena health. 2018 Feb;**14**. Available from: https://www.athenahealth.com/insight/healthcare-future-female

[41] Piraro D, Howath W. Doctor with reflex hammer and clown on exam table. Online image. King Features Syndicate; 2018. Available from: https://comicskingdom.com/bizarro/2018-02-24 [Accessed: 29 December 2018]

[42] Farraj R, Baron JH. Why do hospital doctors wear white coats? Journal of the Royal Society of Medicine [Internet]. 1991 Jan;**84**(1):43. DOI: 10.1177/014107689108400116

[43] Eriksson N. Doctor misinterprets x-ray. Online image. King Features Syndicate; 2017. Available from: http://comicskingdom.com/search?page=14&q=doctor&utf8=✓ [Accessed: 29 December 2018]

[44] Hoest B, Reiner J. What you have is curable Mr. Lockhorn. Online image. King Features Syndicate; 2017. Available from: http://lockhorns.com/comics/december-1-2017/ [Accessed: 29 December 2018]

[45] Price H. Modern medicine. Online image. King Features Syndicate; 2018. Available from: http://rhymeswithorange.com/comics/january-16-2018/ [Accessed: 29 December 2018]

[46] Cohn N, Murthy B, Foulsham T. Meaning above the head: combinatorial constraints on the visual vocabulary of comics. Journal of Cognitive Psychology [Internet]. 2016 May;**28**(5):559-574. DOI: 10.1080/20445911.2016.1179314

[47] Farinella M. Of microscopes and metaphors: Visual analogy as a scientific tool. The Comics Grid: Journal of Comics Scholarship [Internet]. 2018;**8**(1). DOI: 10.16995/cg.130

[48] Grice HP. Logic and conversation. In: Cole P, Morgan JL, editors. Syntax and Semantics, Speech Acts. Vol. 1975, 3. New York: Academic Press; 1975. pp. 41-58

[49] Fazio LK, Brashier NM, Payne BK, Marsh EJ. Knowledge does not protect against illusory truth. Journal of Experimental Psychology: General [Internet]. 2015 Oct;**144**(5):993-1002. DOI: 10.1037/xge0000098